THE ONES I CARRY

TARA DUFFY

Published by Shifted Ground Press

Pittsburgh, Pennsylvania

ISBN: 979-8-9957619-0-7

Cover design by Chris Rychter

Interior design by Tara Duffy

This is a work of creative nonfiction. Some names and identifying details have been changed to protect privacy.

Printed in the United States of America

Contact: shiftedgroundllc@gmail.com

For those who let me walk beside them.

Some moments don't end. They keep moving inside us.

AUTHOR'S NOTE

This book began as a collection of moments—scribbled in margins, typed in the dark, whispered into the spaces between infusions, shifts, and bedtime stories. I didn't set out to write a memoir. I set out to remember.

To remember the patients who let me in.

To remember the stories that changed me.

To remember the way grief and grace often arrive hand in hand.

Over the years, I've had the privilege of walking alongside people at their most vulnerable, when the veil between life and death thins and what matters most rises to the surface. These stories are not just about dying. They are about living—fiercely, honestly, and with open hearts.

Writing this book has been an act of presence. A way to hold onto what I've learned and offer it forward. I hope these pages remind you of your own moments—the ones that shimmer quiet or burn loud, the ones that ache, the ones that changed you.

To my patients: Thank you for letting me witness your lives.

To my family: Thank you for your wild, honest aliveness—

the heartbeat beneath every page.
To the reader: Thank you for walking with me.
May we all keep showing up.
May we all keep watching for the light.
—Tara

SEPTEMBER 2015

CHAUTAUQUA LAKE, NY

SMALL TALK

I was supposed to be making small talk, but the sky stole me. Blue and orange spilled across the horizon, clouds drifting beyond its edge. The setting sun cast its last glimmers, the water below lighting up like a painted canvas. In its glow, the light shifted, and the moment went with it.

The September breeze chilled my bare limbs as summer faded. I leaned into Dave, his arms wrapping around me. He looked dapper in his suit and tie, sleeves casually rolled to the elbows, his forearms radiating a warmth that felt older than our six months together.

Around us, everyone was in their Sunday best, drinks in hand, circling the safe edges of conversation: "Isn't the weather gorgeous?" "Time flies, doesn't it?" "What do you do for work?" At a wedding full of strangers, I slipped into the same rhythm.

"I'm an oncology nurse," I said, the words landing heavier than I meant. The mood tilted. Silence loomed. I sipped my water and hoped the funny guy beside me might rescue the moment.

"Uplifting," he said, his sarcasm cutting through the pause.

"That's usually the reaction," I faltered, flushing red, my

nervous smile doing little to mask the discomfort. I'd answered honestly at a wedding, of all places. Three years into oncology nursing, I was still wading through the muddy waters of how to bring my profession into small talk.

It's always the same.

The pause, the flicker of unease. The way the air shifts the moment oncology is spoken aloud, the way eyes drop for half a beat. I considered skirting the question to spare the mood. But I never did. Maybe it's because I didn't believe cancer was all tears and sadness.

"It actually can be," I heard myself say. Heads turned. "I find my patients very much alive."

The mood lifted, faces softening, waiting for me to say more. But I didn't because I didn't know how.

How do I convey the patient who gets outside for the first time in a month and cannot stop smiling, the son who visits his father's bedside after years of estrangement, or the young woman writing her own eulogy?

How do I describe the laughter that fills a room during a head-shaving party, the joy of dancing with a patient during a bell-ringing celebration, or the patient-turned-friend who teaches me the raw edges of life?

Some things don't fit neatly into small talk.

But they deserve to be told.

PART I

2012—ROCHESTER, NY

17 MINUTES

I walked the half mile to my final nursing school requirement: Capstone, a 100-hour clinical internship shadowing an experienced nurse in the emergency room. The walk was my stillness before the rapid-fire rhythm inside.

Nothing in the ER stopped moving. Antiseptic hung in the air. Pumps beeped. The intercom barked. Stretchers rushed past. It was relentless. A blur of motion and sound. A cycle of urgency. So far from the quiet, grounded places where I usually felt most like myself.

I'd already secured a job in the ER, and with limited spots available, getting one felt like an achievement. So I took it.

Patients came and went. Turnover was the goal. Get them in, get them out. It was efficient, but it felt like we were only skimming the surface of people's lives. My supervisor kept me moving. "Meet them, treat them, and street them," he'd say. But the work fell short of anything meaningful.

So, one evening I asked him, "Do you like getting to know patients?"

"Nope," he said. "I don't want to know anything about them

—not their names, not their stories. That's why I work in the ER." He stood and walked away.

He may have been in the right place, but I wasn't sure I was.

Around 2 a.m., a man stumbled off the street in full cardiac arrest. He was drenched in sweat, reeking of urine. I cycled through rounds of chest compressions, switching off with another nurse, his ribs cracking beneath my hands. We never got his heart to beat on its own. After 17 minutes, the time of death was called.

The only thing I knew about this man was where his ribs met his sternum.

THE SPARK

When the dust settled, I asked if anyone knew his story. No one answered. Or maybe no one wanted to. I stood there, hands still tingling, wondering how many stories we lost this way. I never wanted to just treat bodies. I wanted to know the people inside them.

There was one brief elective rotation before I finished nursing school: a two-day stint on the bone marrow transplant unit. I signed up at the suggestion of a classmate.

On this floor, cancerous bone marrow is obliterated with chemotherapy and replaced with healthy cells from a donor. Patients stay in isolation for weeks, sometimes months. I was there for two 12-hour shifts.

That's when I met Ron. He was prepping for his transplant, pale and exhausted, but his eyes sparked with a kind of spunk.

"What do you do for work?" I asked, wrapping a blood pressure cuff around his bicep.

"Mechanic—been one since I was yay high," he said, motioning to his knee with his calloused hands. "Fixing things. And I race."

"Race?" I asked.

"Yeah. You ever been in a racecar?"

I shook my head.

Ron leaned in, his face lit up. "Behind the wheel, everything fades—bills, worries, heartaches. It's just you, the road, and the engine's heartbeat. Especially in a machine you've built yourself."

"You build racecars?"

"Built a car. A boat. And an airplane."

"Wow. Which one do you love most?"

"Racing," he said instantly. "The boat was slow. The plane was a thrill, but once it flew, the magic faded. I was just floating." He paused, then grinned. "But my lap record—the fastest of all time—that's my real pride."

"I wish he built birdhouses," his wife said, never looking up from her knitting.

As I left that day, something shifted, a quiet click inside me, like a door I hadn't realized was waiting to open until that moment. I didn't know what to call it yet, only that I wanted to feel what Ron felt: purpose and transcendence. I'd always loved hearing people's stories. Ron made me want to stay long enough to learn them.

The next morning, I called the nurse recruiter.

"I don't want the ER position," I said.

She sounded surprised. "But you don't have another job."

Finding me a job was her job.

"I want to work in oncology," I told her.

There was a long pause.

"Okay," she finally said. "Let's get you an interview then."

It felt like a small decision at the time, just another phone call.

STRONG

At thirty, I started my first nursing job in Rochester, New York, on the Hematology/Oncology unit of the Wilmot Cancer Center at Strong Memorial Hospital—a name that felt aspirational at the time. In my badge photo, I'm smiling like someone who has no idea what's ahead. It was a wide, hopeful smile. I didn't know it yet, but this job would teach me how to live with grief without letting it hollow me out. It was a leukemia and lymphoma unit—acute myeloid leukemia (AML), acute lymphocytic leukemia (ALL)—the kinds of cancers that kept people with us long enough to feel like family.

A couple months in, I told my parents about a patient who had passed. My dad asked, "Isn't that hard, dealing with all that dying?"

It was. For the most part, I was numb. I wasn't processing the grief so much as tucking it away.

Six months in, I tried to get a handle on my coping skills. I took up hot yoga, hoping to sweat it all out. I started journaling, trying to trap my feelings between the lines. Still, the heaviness made me wonder if I wasn't cut out for oncology, as if grief meant failure. As if strength and sorrow couldn't coexist.

I worked with nurses who broke down in tears, sometimes over one sentence or memory. Our leukemia patients faced long, grueling journeys, and happy endings felt rare. A seasoned nurse told me remission felt like the exception, not the rule. It wasn't a statistic, but it was the floor sentiment.

Every day felt like climbing a steep, slippery incline, knowing some patients wouldn't make it to the next ledge. People suggested easier jobs. Management encouraged us to "stay busy" to keep our minds off the losses. It was the American way: keep moving, keep upright, keep the feelings from leaking out sideways.

I did that sometimes. But with every passing patient, I started to let the feelings in. Not to drown in them, just to stop hiding from what they meant.

"Yes, Dad, the loss is hard." It was the best I could answer. I still didn't understand the full magnitude of the career ahead.

"Well, stick with it," he said. "Maybe it'll get easier."

Maybe he meant I'd grow. Or maybe he meant I'd grow numb to it.

Either way, doing hard things wasn't about them becoming easy—it was about growing strong enough to hold them. The days and nights, the ups and downs, the ache and the awe began to feel like a fuller way of living.

I didn't expect this job to be all rainbows and sunshine. But I believed the stories mattered. Slowly, patient by patient, the work began to feel different.

REMEMBERING THE SKY

The jackhammers were pounding again, dust drifting across the sidewalk—a daily disruption I'd learned to tune out. It should've been a sight for sore eyes, but I'd stopped looking, pressing my hands over my ears as I hurried past.

Inside, the fluorescent lights hummed. The air smelled of antiseptic and overcooked vegetables. I walked the familiar hallway, scanning whiteboards and monitors, bracing for the weight of the day.

Annie's smile caught mine. I hadn't seen it in weeks.

"Did you finally get outside today?" I asked, surprised by the lightness in her face.

Annie had been asking for weeks. First, she'd asked to attend her niece's wedding, but doctors denied the request—her immune system was too low. Then, insurance informed her that if she left, she'd have to pay for her entire hospital stay. "I feel like I'm jailed," she told me once. After that, her asks grew simpler. She just wanted fresh air.

"I did. It was greeeaat," she sighed, stretching the word like a song.

She beamed as I wrote my name on the whiteboard. Her

bald head was tucked under a knit cap. She'd been in the same room for over a month, tethered to monitors, IV poles, and the hospital bed.

"Where did you get to go?" I asked.

"Just out front," she said matter-of-factly.

It was just the construction site, and I felt a flicker of dismay.

"I forgot the sky was so big," she whispered.

Her wonder pulled something awake in me.

I couldn't remember the last time I'd noticed it. I stood beside her, unsure if I should speak, so I didn't.

Annie exhaled deeply, her shoulders relaxing as if the memory itself was medicinal. She told me how the nurse wheeled her out, bundled in blankets. The crisp fall air greeted her like an old forgotten friend. She closed her eyes and tilted her face toward the sun, letting it kiss her skin. She'd removed her knit cap, and the breeze had touched her bare head for the first time. "It tickled," she giggled. And, for a moment, she forgot about the weight of her diagnosis.

"I could smell fall through the leaves," she said. "And the wind, it felt like it was knocking the dust right off my soul."

I pictured her sitting there, surrounded by dust and noise, yet completely transported.

I found myself smiling, too. I wanted to say something worthy, but her words carried more than mine ever could, so I let the silence hold us. Because sometimes silence is the only way to honor a moment that feels like grace. She remembered the sky. And I remembered why I was falling for oncology.

A BLUEBIRD DAY

The morning I met Maya, six inches of fresh powder covered the ground. I've always loved snow days—the excuse to be a kid again, to slow down, to play, to forget the rules for a while. But with a 12-hour shift ahead, it felt like Mother Nature was teasing me. I threw on my scrubs, bitter. Even my dog, Rocky, looked disappointed we couldn't enjoy the snow.

As I trudged through the beautiful fluff, I imagined a mountainside waiting for someone to glide through the powder. The sun broke through the skyline, bouncing light off the snowbanks. A bluebird day, the kind I hated wasting at work. I wore my sulk into the hospital.

Maya coined it before I did.

"A bluebird day," she said, shimmying upright in her hospital bed.

"You're a skier," I said, half asking.

"Sure am. I'll be back out there next season."

"Great attitude."

She shrugged. "It could always be worse, right?" Her grin was mischievous, too grounded to be passive-aggressive, but it still hit me low and sharp.

Maya was twenty-seven—close to my own age, but she had the kind of spirit that made her seem both ageless and ancient. Like Annie, she was undergoing 7+3 induction, a chemo regimen that wipes out the bone marrow to kill leukemia cells. The hope was remission. Patients stay at least a month, sometimes longer, depending on success.

I noticed my surroundings for the first time—not just the vitals or the chart, but the room itself, the way it held her. Maya's room looked like an elementary school explosion: cards taped to the wall in Crayola scrawl, stick figures so happy they seemed ready to lift off the wall. By the window stood a guitar and a pair of Merrell hiking boots. I could tell a lot about a person by their shoes. I owned the same pair.

"I'm learning how to play," she said, noticing me noticing.

"That is great," I said, thinking of my own guitar, collecting dust.

"A friend taught me the basics."

I smiled. "Let me hear you play."

Maya jumped up with a limber stride, IV pole in tow, and grabbed the guitar. A few brunette strands fell from her head onto the linoleum.

She sat back on the edge of her bed and broke into the opening lines of "The Bare Necessities," her voice light and playful.

"I'm a kindergarten teacher," she said, glancing up, and it all suddenly made sense.

"I sing that for my class every morning. Just trying to remind them of what matters."

I felt awe soften my insides. The snow-day grump, the envy, all of it melted in her voice.

"I love your creativity," I said, as she gently placed the guitar on her lap. A few more strands of hair slipped from beneath her cap. She adjusted her gown with a practiced grace, learning to move with tubes and lines—a choreography no twenty-seven-year-old should have to master.

"What's your creative outlet?" Maya looked up, her gaze curious.

"I like to write," I admitted. "Though I don't do it much now," I added, wondering why not.

"You should," she said, a wry smile playing on her lips. "Write about the snow day you missed out on." Her mischievous gaze lingered, and I wondered if this kindergarten teacher was schooling me.

A THOUSAND TINY PIVOTS

I wasn't counting my blessings. I had the privilege of showing up, clocking in, doing my job, but I carried a restlessness I couldn't name. A selfish pull I kept trying to outrun.

I felt unsettled. I had a boyfriend who bored me and a job that rattled me. I lived for snow days, hikes, and last-minute road trips. Commitment made me itchy, plans breakable, excuses easy, a whole life built on escape routes. My world revolved around small comforts that barely buffered the loneliness I never admitted to.

But with each patient, something quiet in me shifted. Their honesty, their dreams, their courage—these weren't just stories I heard. They were quiet recalibrations, steady and unassuming. It was happening beneath the surface long before I understood it. Patient by patient, I grew humbler.

I came to work bone-tired, counting the hours to sleep. Benny woke me in a different way.

It was 6 a.m. The room smelled faintly of antiseptic and stale coffee. He caught me mid-yawn, scanning his morning meds. The third 12-hour night shift in a row. I was ready to go horizontal.

"Don't work so hard," he shouted like he was scolding someone in the next room. Even sick, Benny sat upright with defiance. His mediport peeked just below his collarbone, a lifeline for chemo, but he radiated strength, almost confrontational.

"Don't," he barked again.

I held up my hands. "Okay, I won't." I wasn't about to argue—it wasn't really about me.

"Did you just wake up, Benedict?" I asked, eyeing his 6 a.m. energy.

"Benny," he said, waving off the question. "I'm Benedict when I'm in trouble."

I smiled. His humor was sharp, almost angry, but somehow still charming.

"You have a beautiful smile—you married?" he asked.

"Easy over there," came a voice from across the room. His wife sat up on the futon, blankets in a heap. "Don't go dancing without me now."

I smiled, and she caught it.

"Well?" She gave a little wave, urging me on.

"I'm not married," I blushed, the answer too familiar.

"Boyfriend? Girlfriend?" she asked, sincere.

"Boyfriend."

"He a good guy?" Benny stared me down, reading something between the lines.

"He is," I said, hesitating.

The pause hung there. They noticed.

Darren was kind and steady but starting to feel more like a placeholder. We met hiking with our dogs, a serendipitous moment that felt destined for more than it was becoming.

Benny didn't know the details, but he saw the truth anyway.

"Come on," he said. "Don't settle. Life's too short for that shit."

"We'll see," I said, a nervous chuckle slipping out. And I heard my own hesitance.

"What do you mean we'll see?!" His stare held steady, challenging but clear. "Do you like the guy or not?"

I wanted to laugh it off, move on, blame it on exhaustion. But their words hit harder than I expected. I'd asked myself these questions before, just never out loud.

"Girl," Benny's wife jumped in, wrapping a hoodie around her shoulders. She walked toward me with a sway and tossed her arm through mine. "Come to Zumba with me. We'll find someone who lights you up."

I laughed, half uncomfortable, half grateful. They were strangers, yet they saw me more clearly than I saw myself. I didn't go to Zumba, but I started listening more closely to the questions I kept dodging.

HALFWAY THROUGH

"I heard once that every ended relationship," Maya said slowly, as if pulling the thought up from somewhere deep, "should've ended halfway through its length."

"Really?" I nodded, thinking of the ones I'd dragged out far too long. "That actually sounds about right," I chuckled, trying not to think about the one I was still in.

"I think it is for most of us." She had recently ended a relationship that had spanned from high school through early adulthood. "It ended for several reasons—mostly, he bored me to tears."

She shook her head, clearing the last of it away.

"I kept hoping he'd wake up, want to see the world the way I do. But he loved his video games. I want someone who can sit under the stars and wonder how they light up." Her eyes went wide, lit with something childlike.

"That's brave," I said. "Most of us stay long past the ending."

"It wasn't easy," she admitted. "But then again, nothing worth anything ever is."

Outside, a weak sun was struggling to break through the gray sky, its faint light touching her face as if it, too, was holding on to some shred of hope. Empathy swept through me like a full-moon tide. I wished I were more like her.

A first love behind her, a body weakened by illness, adventures on hold—and still, she believed in starlight.

Maybe hope is the last thing illness can touch. Or maybe illness illuminates it.

The room stilled, her words hanging in the air. I couldn't remember the last time I looked at the stars with wonder. Somewhere along the way, I'd stopped looking up.

WHERE IT BEGAN

I visited Maya because I thought she needed company. I imagined time dragged on behind those walls, and Maya had only one steady visitor, Carly, a family friend. She never knew her mother. Her father came infrequently. Her brother was overseas.

As Maya wore down from chemo, our conversations thinned. In that quiet, I understood something I hadn't before: while I thought I was caring for Maya, she'd been quietly filling a void I didn't know I had.

Early into my night shift, Maya's constant, Carly, found me sipping my coffee.

"Hey, Tara, Maya has been asking for you."

It had been over a week since I last visited her.

"Oh hey, Carly, how is she?"

"Well, stop by. She'd love to see you." Her lips flattened, as if they wanted to smile but couldn't quite get there.

The room was packed with friends in their twenties, warm and loud. They greeted me with firm handshakes and hugs. I did my best to soften my stiff embrace. Someone handed me a bowl of turkey chili and thanked me for being such a great nurse. I didn't know if they said that to everyone who entered their circle, but I was learning that presence is its own kind of care.

Within minutes, the most boisterous of the bunch, surfer hair, full smile, emerged from the bathroom holding a razor in one hand and a pile of blond curls in the other. Half his head looked like a cue ball. The room erupted.

Maya clapped from her bed as I looked at the strands of hair scattered across the sheets. We'd talked about shaving her head. Hair loss was always hard, especially for women. Hair says something in this culture. Sometimes everything.

She stood slowly, tossing a towel around her shoulders, fists clenched, elbows bent. "My turn," she said. Her eyes brimmed with tears, love and loss rising at the same time.

That night, three guys, one girl, and Maya all shaved their heads. Carly did Maya's, one clean stroke down the center. She left it that way long enough to do the chicken dance. By the end of the show, my eyes were wet too. Happy tears, sad ones, the whole mix. I couldn't think of anywhere else I'd rather be.

As her friends began to leave, hugs all around, I stepped in one more time before the night ended.

"Your head looks great," I said, a little awkward. I'd heard other nurses say it. But I was still learning the language of these moments, and when silence was the kinder choice.

She brushed off the compliment, burning past the small talk. "How's the writing going?"

I paused.

"There's been no writing," I admitted.

But Maya's glacial stare cut through the excuses stacking in my throat. It was the moment I knew I couldn't keep not writing.

"Actually...I think I've got myself a story."

A smile rose to her face, brighter now for the hair that no longer framed it.

The idea fluttered in, light, and I had to write it down before it flew away. Six months into nursing, my storytelling began with Maya, somewhere around midnight. It started with the snow day I missed and the friendship I made.

And in that space, I began to discover what mattered.

TINY

His smile was wry, a bit of mischief in its rise.

"I can tell you are a troublemaker," he teased as I asked about his coffee. According to other nurses, this was a sore subject. Mike was a tough critic.

"Coffee's still terrible," he muttered, shaking his head.

He'd rung the call bell the day before, ranting about it until I made him a fresh pot.

"Can I make you another pot?" I offered.

"Okay, I'll take you for the day…" He grinned, reading my badge. "Ta-Ra."

"Yes—I'm Tara," I said, smiling.

"Help yourself," he said. He'd caught my hungry eyes scanning his tray of untouched fruit.

"No, I'm fine, but thank you." I chuckled, embarrassed to be caught.

"Here, help me out," he said, tossing me an orange. "They tell me to eat more fruit. Eat it here so I can show them the remnants." He laughed hard at his idea.

I peeled it immediately, the citrus mist mingling with the scent of coffee grounds.

"We owe ourselves a proper introduction," I smiled, scanning his chart. "Do you go by Mike?"

He grinned, mischief returning.

"Tiny."

He let out a belly laugh, loving his own joke. Mike was 51, built like a linebacker—his hospital bed was the only thing tiny about him.

"You liked that one?"

"Very much," I said between chuckles.

His light drew me in. Plump and bald, there was something grounding about his presence.

I eventually completed his assessment. The laughter delayed us, but those endorphins felt like the perfect start to my stretch of 12-hour shifts.

When I re-entered his room an hour later, he said, "What took you so long?"

His tone had shifted.

"Did we have something set?" I asked, confused.

"No. I need some water," he said, flat.

He didn't speak again, so I did.

"Why didn't you call me?" I motioned toward the bell. He'd been quick to use it yesterday.

He looked me straight in the eye.

I waited.

He let the silence stretch.

"Lazy," he said, then burst into a belly laugh.

Mike always laughed before the punchline, he thought he was hilarious. And he was. His humor was easy, the kind that made you feel lighter without trying.

His room held three large canvases of his boys—between five and 10, judging by the gap-toothed smiles. Their eyes sparkled, each picture a story. I imagined sticky fingers, couch forts, wild laughter. He didn't need water. He needed company.

He caught me staring. "They're my *why*," he said, voice catching.

I offered a smile. "I bet. Tell me about these handsome guys."

His face softened. "That's Mickey. Loves fishing, just like me. Thinks he's hilarious."

"Like his dad," I said, and he nodded with a chuckle.

"Careful," he teased. "You're gonna make me think I'm actually funny."

"And Cal is the artist, always drawing something. And Mason. Doesn't stop moving. Either a hundred miles an hour or completely passed out."

He stared at the canvases. "I miss them." His voice dropped. "It's hard to realize what we have...when we have it." He swallowed. "I just...I'd give anything to hear them fighting over a ball, or see their muddy footprints across the hardwood."

His words settled beneath my collarbone.

"It's hard to appreciate the little things while we're in them," I said.

His eyes shimmered. "We think we have all the time in the world, but we don't. Never did."

I reached out and patted his shoulder. He relaxed beneath my hand. I felt awkward, but he didn't.

"Most of us take our time here for granted. Give yourself some grace."

A bittersweet smile crept in. "Well, *don't*, Tara."

We laughed, uneasy but honest.

"You have a family, Tara?"

I shook my head. "No, I don't."

"Yet." He winked.

I could hear the clock ticking on the wall as we sat beside one another.

"When you have kids of your own," Mike said, eyes drifting, "slow down with them. Try to soak it all in. Don't brush past their curious questions, even when life pulls at you from all sides." He sighed. "Soak it all in, all of it."

His words hovered. I nodded, letting their weight sink in.

"Will do, Mike," I said. But he didn't hear me. He was somewhere else.

I carried his words with me, tucked between my badge and my heart. I didn't know it then, but I'd return to them, and to him, more than once.

"OKAY."

Somewhere between dog walks and beers, Darren started talking about children.

"I always thought it would happen for me," he said on numerous occasions, a belief I shared.

I just wasn't sure it would happen for us.

We were hiking with the dogs at a favorite local park. The incline was sharp, and ice and snow lined the trail. The dogs bounded ahead, their paws kicking up snow sprays as my boots crunched against the frozen trail. Frost clung to the edges of my jacket, and each breath hung visible in the cold air.

"Same," I admitted. "But I've never felt in a rush for children either."

I loved caring for my dog and wanted motherhood someday, but I wasn't sure Darren was the right partner for that journey. I wasn't convinced Rochester was my forever place—if such a place even existed.

If I loved him, maybe it wouldn't matter where we lived. That's what people said love could do.

"Move in with me," he said as we reached the peak. "That will be a good test for us."

I took a deep breath, wondering if relationships were supposed to need tests. My lease ended in a month, and saying yes felt less like a choice and more like a quiet surrender to convenience. I remembered my friend's advice: make decisions from a position of strength, not weakness.

And yet, weakness was easier.

"Okay," slipped out of my mouth. "We can see how it goes," I said with a reluctance I ignored.

THE ORANGE

Patient conversations had begun to shift something in me.

I didn't always notice it in the moment, but afterward—walking back to the nurses' station, peeling off gloves, scribbling notes—I felt lighter. Their honesty cut through the numbness I'd been carrying, the routines I'd mistaken for purpose.

I stepped into Mike's room, already bracing for whatever version of him I'd get that day.

"I was hoping I'd get you again, Tara—I need help with these oranges," he said, eyes lighting up as he gestured to a pile nestled between cookie crumbs.

"Oh good, I'm here to help, Mike."

"Peel them in here so I can tell everyone I ate my orange," he laughed. A citrus missile flew toward my head. I caught it, inches from my temple.

"Whoa—good hands." He looked almost disappointed, like he'd hoped it would hit me.

"Well, you threw it at my head!"

"Who knew quick reflexes would come in handy with a cancer patient?" he said, his laugh booming through the room. I couldn't help but laugh too.

"How are those handsome boys?" I asked, nodding toward the pictures on his wall.

The question hung in the air, more an invitation than a distraction.

Mike leaned back in his bed, his smile softening as his gaze landed on the photos of his sons.

"You know, Tara," he said quietly, "I used to rush through everything. Now I just want them to slow down. Stay little a little longer."

He rubbed his thinning hair. "But it's funny…time, it just… slips by." His voice faltered. "It's all just a blip, really."

A lump rose in my throat, catching me off guard.

His words stayed with me long after I left the room, orange in hand. I was assigned to Mike less often in the weeks that followed, but I still popped in—to catch a story, fine-tune a harmless prank, or bring a fresh cup of coffee. He always accepted, slipping me a specially saved orange on my way out.

"Tara saves Tiny," he'd say with a smirk. "You know I need help with this fruit."

Excuse or not, it was a thoughtful gesture. And somewhere between the banter and bedside rituals, Mike had become someone I looked forward to each shift.

The zesty orange aroma lingered, like Mike's laughter. And something in me stayed lighter because of him.

THE BEREAVEMENT TRAY

"I need a bereavement tray," I overheard my charge nurse, Callie, say as she pointed toward Tiny's room. It was my first day back after a stretch off.

"He passed?" I managed, knowing a bereavement tray meant an assortment of snacks for the grieving family.

"He did. It was unexpected," she said, giving me the brief nod nurses use when there's no time to go any deeper.

I fought the frog that crept into my throat. My eyes welled, and I tried to collect myself as I stepped into Mike's room. My throat burned from swallowing the emotions threatening to spill out. The room felt too quiet, the absence of his laugh heavy in the air.

The wall where his sons once smiled back was bare. Their absence hit harder than the quiet. The lifelong questions his boys would carry with them—how would they make sense of a world without their father's steady presence? Who would teach them to shave or how to laugh at nothing?

The day blurred into tasks, each one a place to hide the grief. Whenever it surfaced, I pushed it down and pressed onward.

At the end of the day, walking the unit, I noticed an

untouched tray of goodies in my peripheral vision. It sat on one of our nurses' stations, Mike's bereavement tray, stacked with treats. I approached it.

And there it stood, almost transcendent: a lone orange cresting the pile of snacks.

BENNY

When I returned to the unit after sleeping the day away, Benny looked like he'd aged a decade. The man who barked at dawn now lay folded into the bed, his edges dulled by something heavier than exhaustion.

"I'm miserable here, Tara. I need to leave."

The words came flat, his face glazed with a kind of emotional weariness I hadn't seen in him before.

He'd just completed induction with 7+3 and was bracing for consolidation, but both his body and spirit were worn. Hope is hard to hold when you feel like hell. Benny had been trapped in the same hospital bed for weeks.

"What's going on?" I asked, scooting closer on my stool.

Benny let out a long breath.

"Just go on vacation. Do more of what you love. Find someone who excites you. Look at me." He gestured to the bed. "This isn't living. I worked hard all my life, and now I'm here. I may never leave."

A hospital bed can become a vault for buried truths—grief, guilt, the ache of unlived days.

"Do you enjoy your work, Benny?" I asked, instantly unsure if the question would help or hurt.

He met my eyes, hollowed.

"Enjoy? I work seven days a week. It's just what I do."

I sank back on the stool, wishing I could take the question back.

"I watched my kids grow up. That should've taught me to slow down," he said, voice catching.

Slow down sounded simple, but I didn't know how to do it. Not yet.

"This bed is terrible," he shouted through a smirk.

I chuckled. "Yeah, it doesn't look great."

"It's terrible," he said again, a half-smile tugging at his mouth. Then, silence.

Sometimes the days blur, one into the next, until you look up and realize how much time has slipped. I wasn't sure when I was last fully awake.

Benny took a shaky breath.

"I'd love to rewind the tape," he said. "My work...it became everything. It paid the bills."

I let him speak, even as it hurt to watch regret gnaw at him. I knew how self-talk could turn on you—medicine one day, poison the next.

"I'm sorry, Benny," I said, the words small but all I had.

He shook his head. "I feel like my time's running out."

None of us knew if Benny would ever leave the hospital.

"Just don't work so hard," he added. "And find someone who lights you up."

I blushed, caught off guard by the turn in conversation.

"Okay, I will, Benny," I said—if not to comfort him, then maybe to believe it myself.

His expression softened.

"Nina is the love of my life."

She was at a Zumba class. She didn't leave the hospital much, just for fresh clothes and Zumba.

"I know I'm lucky," he said. "You will be too. Trust it."

He placed a fist to his chest and winked.

I smiled back, unsure what it was I was trusting.

DOGFISH AND DOWNWARD DOG

After my third 12-hour shift, the kind that leaves you hollowed out and buzzing, I bought a four-pack of Dogfish Head IPA. I wasn't a heavy drinker, ever. Just the occasional beer with friends, light and easy. But this wasn't that kind of night. These were hard feelings, not social ones.

The rental house I shared with two nursing school friends had a porch swing bed, my sweet spot for journaling. I stretched my legs across Rocky, popped the cap, and let the scent of hops mingle in the breeze. The first sip tasted bittersweet, loosening something tight inside me. By the time I stood, a bottle was empty, and so was the weight I'd carried. Or so I wanted to believe.

The next night, I passed the fridge and felt the pull of the Dogfish Heads, promising their gentle hush. My resolve wobbled. It startled me how quickly comfort could blur into numbing. I grabbed Rocky's leash and walked off the pull. I didn't want to become someone who needed to forget to keep going.

The next day I tried yoga.

There, I began to reclaim something. Through motion and

breath, I found a rhythm between holding on and letting go. In downward dog, the weight I'd stored in my shoulders began to unwind.

I started to crave yoga: The sweat, the stretch, the stillness inside the flow. It became the kind of release that didn't ask me to forget.

It helped me stay.

And write it all down.

WHITE CHRISTMAS

I wish I could bottle gratitude and sip it as needed, like a good wine. Short of that, I wanted my time to be quality. But even after my steady diet of inpatient wisdom, I was toddler-like, dragging my feet into work.

It was Christmas Day, 11 a.m. to 11 p.m.: The shift no one wanted.

"Doesn't get much worse than that," my best friend from college, Meg, said over the phone as I trudged into the Christmas shift.

I agreed, "Sure doesn't," forgetting how often I walked past suffering.

But actually, it could get worse.

Ally was 48. Diagnosed late Christmas Eve. Paralyzed from the waist down. A spinal tumor had stolen her movement in a single night.

She smiled as she introduced her "pack": Adult children, nieces, nephews, sisters, in-laws, and a husband whose devotion was immediately evident. They greeted me with waves and warmth that made the room feel lighter. In the corner, someone had assembled an impromptu Christmas tree resembling

Charlie Brown's, with handwritten bulbs dangling as ornaments. It was beautiful. A gesture of defiance, maybe. Or hope.

"Welcome to the pack, Tara," Ally said, her cheeks pale, but there was a light in her eyes that made the room feel less clinical, more human. She turned her attention to an ornament in her lap, scribbling on its blank surface with a Sharpie. Then she handed it to me.

"Go ahead, hang that up for me."

The room quieted as I stepped toward their small tree. The bulb read:

Happiness, not in another place but this place, not in another hour but this hour.

"Did you come up with that?" I asked.

"I did," she said, "but I can't take credit. It's Whitman. I'm trying to fill this room with good energy. God knows I need it now."

Her voice dipped for just a moment. I wondered if she'd always lived like this, attuned to the moment, or if that clarity came only with her diagnosis.

"Come back for dinner," she said. "We've got plenty."

I did. The whole nursing staff did. Home-cooked food that smelled like hope. We piled in and ate like family.

At shift change, I said goodbye to Ally.

"Dinner was so nice, Ally. Thank you."

"It's the least I could do for all of you stuck here today," she replied.

"It's actually been a great Christmas," I said. "You made it more than work."

Her room was quiet now. Her pack gone. She opened her arms, and I stepped in. We'd just met 12 hours earlier, but the hug made sense. That's how fast some people get under your skin.

"Thank you for everything," she said, her voice cracking.

"It's my pleasure," I replied as tears spilled down her cheeks. Something had broken open.

"What can I do?" I asked, desperate to fix what I couldn't name.

"I'm giving myself some time for self-pity," she said.

Grief with a curfew. What a concept.

Her husband returned, and together we repositioned her legs. No one spoke. Then he traced a finger along her foot.

"Hey! That tickles!" she squealed.

He kept going, tickle-torturing limbs she couldn't move. It was oddly cruel and perfect. Her laughter caught like wildfire. I left on that wave, pillow fights and grace and everything unexpected.

In the elevator, my legs ached. But my heart had been recalibrated. I'd arrived bracing for the kind of Christmas no one wants to work. I left with a family that wasn't mine, and hope that didn't have to be.

The elevator doors opened, and the cold hit me. Outside, the snow shimmered in the moonlight. There's something about snow on Christmas that fills me with promise, like childhood snow days that stretched endlessly or Christmas mornings thick with anticipation. I wondered if other children went to bed satisfied, or a little sad, the way I used to feel when the magic slipped into Christmas night. The collision of anticipation and ache.

Even as a child, I felt both.

DEATH IN THE DOORWAY

"He's still hanging on. His son's on the way," Mira, my coworker, said, raising an eyebrow. "You know that story, right?"

John had just been transferred to our floor the week before. Palliative care was leading his treatment with one goal: comfort. I'd sat with him the shift prior as he drifted between sleep and something deeper. Staff said he hadn't spoken to his son in over a decade. No one knew why. And I was somehow the chosen one to hold the room steady. A dull ache pressed behind my eyes.

"I do." I raised both eyebrows and felt a ripple of nerves. Days like this could undo you.

Mira smiled. "Sorry you're stuck with this doozy of an assignment," she said, drifting toward the door.

"Father Joe knows the situation, call him if needed. And Barb's at the bedside, just in case." It was standard to keep someone close near the end. Barb was our nurse leader.

Mira and I entered the room for bedside report before she clocked out. We did this at every shift change, night nurses signing off, dayshift stepping in. I walked straight into John's bed extension; he was too tall for a standard frame, and the metal bar slammed into my shin. A sharp, stupid pain shot up my leg.

"Easy," Barb whispered.

John didn't move. He lay there motionless, pillows tucked beneath his knees and ankles. Fluid pooled in his legs; his organs were failing. His skin was clammy, yellow with jaundice. Each ragged breath lifted one cheek in uneven rhythm, underscored by a gurgling rasp. I rubbed my shin and blinked back tears. A dying patient and a bum leg—and I was already bracing.

"And that's about all I've got," Mira said with a grin, already halfway out the door. "I gotta get the hell outta here."

John's son arrived like a storm front. As Mira held the door open, he filled the frame, tall, broad, disoriented. Behind him, Mira mouthed "so hot," her humor misplaced. I kept my face neutral. The moment was too charged for levity.

He stood frozen in the doorway, not knowing where to put his arms or his body. His shaggy hair skimmed his collar, and the rumpled suit made him look like a surfer forced into a courtroom. I recognized the way he stood there, unsure where to put his emotion. We stared at each other, equally uncertain.

"Hi, I'm Tara, your father's nurse . . ."

He stared at me blankly, and for a second I wasn't sure I'd gotten it right.

"Sorry, you are?" I asked, stumbling.

"I'm Cameron. He's my dad. I heard he doesn't have much time."

He offered his hand to shake, but his gaze never left the bed. His face had gone a shade paler, his eyes wide with something between fear and disbelief.

"Here, have a seat," I said, sliding a chair behind his knees. I wasn't equipped for a reunion like this.

"You can talk to him," Barb said, stepping in.

My hands were balled so tight my nails cut into my palms. Father Joe arrived. My hands unclenched. My breath did too.

Barb stayed at Cameron's side, steadying him through the emotional weight in the room. Cameron stood, towering over the bed, shoulders set like armor, but his jaw trembled. His eyes brimmed. I wondered if both men had lived these past ten years alone in different ways.

"You can tell him you love him," Father Joe said.

I felt like I was intruding on something sacred.

Cameron nodded, then reached for his father's hand. The gesture was small, almost childlike. And there it was again, the things we carry too long and say too late.

"I love you, Dad," Cameron said, his voice trembling. Is it easier to say I love you when there's nothing left to lose?

Then a flicker—John's fingers twitched.

"His fingers," Father Joe whispered.

Cameron looked up, then leaned in, clasping his father's hand.

John's eyes fluttered. "Cameron," he murmured before slipping back under.

Cameron's smile broke halfway, part joy, part grief. Tears streamed unchecked.

"I love you, Dad," he said again, trying to say everything he hadn't said in ten years.

The breaths grew louder, rattling.

Cameron held on. "What's happening?" he asked, panicked.

I froze, words nowhere.

"He's exiting his body," Father Joe said gently. "It's his time now."

The space between each breath lengthened, the rasp turning to hush. We waited.

And then, nothing.

John was gone.

WHEN WE STOP ASKING

John was the first patient I watched die. I hadn't known him long. Just his final few days. But when he passed, a sadness seeped through me. Part of it was for Cameron and for everyone losing a father, a friend, a colleague. But part of it was mine too.

I meet people all the time—in elevators, on chairlifts, in hospital rooms—most forget me as soon as I'm gone. But death is different. It's a full stop. It reminded me not just of everyone I'd lost, but that I would die one day too. And somehow, that truth made even the smallest moments hum with meaning.

"He was the life of every party," Cameron told Barb and me, his jaw clenched. "I know it's hard to imagine now."

"I'd love to hear about him," I offered. I reached for reflection the way I always did when goodbye felt too sharp.

Cameron didn't hesitate.

"He would always play this lion game. I was the kid. He was the lion, roaring and chasing while I shrieked and ran, hysterically laughing." He smiled faintly. "Really, it was the simple things I remember most."

Barb nodded, like she'd heard a hundred versions of this story and held space for each one.

"The tickles," Cameron went on. "The way he'd look me in the eye and listen. The way he never tired of my questions."

His intimidating exterior melted. I could see the ache rising behind his eyes. I wanted to ask why they stopped talking, but it wasn't the question that mattered.

"He always told me to stay curious. To never stop asking questions." He inhaled sharply. "One day, I stopped." His hands trembled as he lifted them to his face.

Barb put an arm around his back, and my hand, stiff and unsure, settled beside hers.

The silence held. Then, slowly, the room began to change.

John was gone. And the world kept moving.

THE MILK TRUCK

After they left with John, I sat for a long time, missing someone who was still alive.

My dad started working on a milk truck at fourteen. He was the fourth of six kids, raised by an alcoholic father who was mostly a shadow in the room. He didn't grow up with much, except for the certainty that he'd do it differently.

By the time I was old enough to notice, my dad had made a career out of court reporting, a job that required precision, silence, and focus. His ethic seeped into the walls of our home. No matter the weather, no matter the hour, he showed up.

He never talked much about the hard details of his childhood, just the great stories. But you could hear it in the way he cleared his throat before difficult conversations, or the way he gave us space when our feelings ran too big for the room. I think he gave us the freedom to feel what he never could.

Sometimes, in the quiet moments between chemo rounds or overnight charting, I'd think about that milk truck. About how much of who we become starts long before we choose it.

THE ONES WHO STAY

Loss sat behind my ribs, a knot I couldn't shake. Mike's especially. I'd started riding to work that summer, the movement helping me shake off the heaviness. I placed my skateboard in my locker and slammed it shut before the blue wheel spun out. Something in me spun with it.

I exhaled and stepped out of the locker room. The room carried that familiar sterile bite. The rhythmic beeping of machines pulled me back into hospital reality, replacing the tree-lined streets from moments before. With each step, the sounds and smells folded back into place, like life after a sudden loss. It just kept rolling forward. I passed Mike's old room. Then Annie's. Then John's.

I turned the corner toward my station, the hallway stretching long ahead of me, illuminated by the dimming lights of the night shift. The familiar routine of the hospital, despite its losses, continued. And yet, I didn't know if I could.

Nurses clustered down the hall, their attention on Brooke. Her sobs were loud, echoing off the walls. Brooke was a coworker who'd started on the floor the same time I did, her face flushed and streaked with tears. I watched the charge nurses shield her as they shuffled her with urgency toward the office. The door closed behind them. The unit buzzed with murmurs, voices low and searching.

"Is she okay?" I asked Mira, who stood by the med cart with her report sheet half-folded.

Mira shrugged, her face drawn. "No clue. No one died today."

Her delivery was blunt in that dry, oddly comforting way she had.

I raised an eyebrow. "Is that our bar now?"

We chuckled, the kind of laugh that tightens your throat.

Night shift carried a strange rhythm—late arrivals, early exits, and a slap-happy thread that ran through the long hours. It was a break from the hustle and demands of the day shift, a space where laughter bubbled up between the grief. Most nights, it was just a lone resident and a band of cool, offbeat nurses who preferred the quiet and the pay bump. I hated what it did to my circadian rhythm almost as much as I loved laughing through the dark.

After checking on my patients, I found Brooke tucked inside a cubicle, her fingers tapping softly against the keyboard. The rest of the unit hummed, but around her, it was still.

"Hey, Brooke, you okay?"

She swiveled, eyes red, brushing a shaky hand through her curls. "Yeah...you saw?"

Embarrassment flushed her face, as if tears were something to apologize for.

"It's okay to cry," I said, words I needed to hear myself. "Sometimes I can't. I just go numb."

"Same. Then it all spills out when I don't ask it to." She hesitated. "This job—it's just so hard sometimes. Patients are here one day, telling me about their daughter's wedding...and then they're gone."

Her voice cracked. "She didn't make it to the wedding." She

wiped her eyes with the back of her hand. "That reminder—it scares me."

I sat on the desk beside her, trying to absorb her grief without pushing it down. Her words lingered between us, heavy and unyielding.

The thought pressed in: Why do we assume we have so many tomorrows?

"My buddy didn't get to see his sons grow up," I said, my voice catching.

Brooke shifted in her chair. "Yeah…I loved Mike, too. That was heartbreaking. Things change so quickly around here."

"I know. Is it just here, though? Or are we just close enough to see how fragile it all is?"

She paused, searching for something. "Good question. I never used to think about dying. Now I do."

I nodded, the truth landing quietly. I thought about the last time I said goodbye to my mom—how I threw in an I love you like a safety net, just in case. I hadn't done that since I was a kid. Something in me had shifted; I felt the weight in every goodbye.

Brooke rose from her chair, her movements steady again, shoulders broad and sure.

"I'm heading to hot yoga."

I nodded, understanding her need to breathe in someone else's ritual. We'd crossed paths there recently, the studio's spiritual messages always eerily timed, like horoscopes vague enough to hit.

"Enjoy," I said, offering half a smile.

She paused in the doorway, shoulders squared. "I thought nursing would be easier." She didn't wait for a reply, and I didn't give one.

GOODBYE FOREVERS

Benny finally entered remission. I spotted him down the hallway, a relaxed smile spreading across his face. When he saw me, he lit up—that same eager, full-body joy I'd come to expect from him.

"I'm allowed to hug you, right?" he asked, arms already open.

"Of course," I said before he pulled me into a bear hug that flushed my face.

"We went on vacation," he beamed. "To the Caribbean. It felt like a dream, Tar." Benny dropped the second syllable of my name somewhere along the way. Just Tar. Like he trimmed the rest to get closer.

He described his wife's childlike euphoria before the trip, the fine restaurants, breathtaking sights, friendships formed. He flipped through photos, hands gesturing with energy. When he finished, his gaze held a softness I hadn't seen before.

"I'm working less." His smile radiated.

"I can tell, Benny."

He seemed lighter. His tone changed. "You break up with the dud yet?" he pressed.

"I did." My voice dipped. I hesitated, tired of goodbyes. "I gave my two weeks; I'm going to be a travel nurse."

Benny frowned, deep lines crinkling his forehead. The space between us shifted.

"Will I ever see you again?"

I hesitated. "I hope so."

His eyebrow lifted the tiniest bit, catching him speechless for the first time since we met. "Ahh, bullshit," he muttered, shaking his head. He pulled me into another bear hug, and I felt his affection in our embrace. When he loosened, he kept his hands on my shoulders, steadying me, as if giving me space to speak.

"Benny, how can I ever forget you?" My voice caught. I smiled, wiping a tear. He had a few of his own, too. He let me go.

"If you're ever in the hood," he said, "come to my restaurant."

"I would love to," I answered, leaving room for hope.

He wrapped me in one more hug, holding on just a bit longer than usual, as if trying to seal the memory for good measure.

When I left Rochester, like every exit, I believed I'd see my friends again. We all say it, forgetting how quickly new routines settle and distance expands.

I hugged Maya goodbye. She had finished consolidation but couldn't bring herself to say the word 'remission,' as if naming it might make it disappear.

We exchanged email addresses and phone numbers. "I can't wait to read your book," she said, her thin arms wrapping around my shoulders. I could feel her bones.

"Keep me posted on everything." I exhaled sharply, stifling the unease.

I grabbed my skateboard from my locker and stepped out of Wilmot Cancer Center for the last time. The brisk fall air met my skin as I pedaled home, carrying a place and stories tucked inside me.

My phone rang. Meg.

“Hey,” I answered, coasting to a stop. The wheels spun. I stared at them, unsure I had the headspace for conversation. I didn’t like how the phone stole my quiet. Or how I let it.

“What’s up? Save any lives today?” her usual greeting.

"Eh, no saved lives, just a whole lot of goodbye forevers."

The words hung in the air. Meg didn’t speak right away.

"Jeez." She paused for a breath. "Meanwhile, my boss lost his shit over a broken Keurig. Ruined everyone's day. Absolute gremlin."

I laughed; Meg could turn anything into a punchline.

"Oh, and Lacoste got engaged. She cried because the diamond wasn't big enough."

She paused, waiting for a reaction I didn't have.

I finally spoke. "Geesh, what different days we had."

I had stories too. Raw, unfiltered ones. One patient wished he had the energy to dance again. Another regretted not eating the brownie when she could taste. One woman longed to brush her hair.

"Yeah, it's no way to live," Meg chuckled, and I was unsure if she was referring to her life or theirs.

I didn't know what Meg actually did all day, but I knew I was around a different breed of people. People who had been stripped of the superficials and forced into a clarity that made the world feel sharper. It was as if they were standing on a cliff's edge where the air was clearer and the views more breathtaking.

And occasionally, just occasionally, I stole a glimpse.

PART II

2014—WASHINGTON, D.C.

SIBLEY MEMORIAL HOSPITAL

THE UNPACKING

In January 2014, I took a 12-week travel nurse assignment at Sibley Memorial Hospital in D.C. The contract came with a studio apartment in Arlington, Virginia. As I unpacked my hoodies, books, and yoga mat, that old ache of dislocation returned. New places felt foreign. Each time I unpacked, I longed for Rochester—once unfamiliar, now home. Growth often came in the lulls, in the still moments, sipping coffee alone at sunrise, wondering if we all saw the same sky. I didn't know it yet, but this was another kind of beginning.

Oncology had rearranged something in me, and I was still figuring out what that meant.

My sister, Shannon—Shan—texted that first night. She knew displacement intimately, a couple months in Ecuador, a solo bike ride down the Pacific Coast, a heli-trip in Alaska. Her excitement about my travel assignment outpaced my own.

"You get to see the world and work—how cool is that?" she wrote.

I could hear the envy tucked inside her enthusiasm. Shan moved often. I didn't. Not really. I liked the idea of rootedness, even when I kept choosing motion.

I'd told Darren my wanderlust was the problem, that I couldn't picture settling down in one place. But really, it was him. We said our goodbyes without plans to keep in touch—clean, final, like a funeral.

"It's pretty cool," I wrote back, trying to believe it.

THE MAESTRO

Sibley Memorial Hospital had a different tempo. The daylight shifts, the weekends off, it felt almost decadent. Patients came in, received their infusions, and returned to their lives: work, school, grocery runs. It was a kind of freedom I hadn't felt in inpatient care, palpable, measured in motion and fresh air.

The infusion room was quiet, pale colors and modern chairs. A single bed sat in the far corner, reserved for patients who were too fatigued to sit or for those labeled "VIP," a designation I never loved. But this was D.C., and plenty of people tried not to be seen.

A few weeks in, I was scanning a patient's chart when my charge nurse leaned in and whispered, "He's VIP." My stomach tensed. I hated the weight those letters carried. VIP meant different rules, different expectations, a hierarchy I never followed. I didn't believe anyone deserved more care than anyone else. I steadied myself and stepped into the room, my nerves tightening under his gaze. As I inserted his IV, he looked up with calm, focused eyes and spoke with an intensity that made my nerves spike. His name was Gustavo.

"No one knows I have cancer."

"Really?"

His chemo regimen would be hard to hide. Hair loss. Fatigue. The kind that flattens a person.

"I'll be at work tomorrow by nine," he said. "People might look at my bald head and wonder, but only my family knows."

I nodded. Most patients leaned on blog updates or email chains, circles of prayer and shared logistics. But support can feel like scrutiny too.

"Why's that?" I asked, instantly regretting it.

His gaze cooled, but he didn't flinch. "Because then they'd pity me. Look at me differently. Treat me like I'm dying." He exhaled slowly. "I don't want to feel like I have cancer. I want to keep doing what I love."

I loved that because it was new to me.

"I'm a maestro."

He was in his eighties. His passion for music unshaken, his body quietly rebellious beneath a crisp sweater and pressed slacks. He told me about his setbacks, teachers, and his earliest concerts. "Your calling finds you," he said when I asked how he'd known. His voice was tinged with memory.

Then he opened his briefcase, pulled out two orchestra tickets, and handed them to me.

"Come."

I smiled, caught off guard. "Thank you. I'd love to."

"Bring someone special," he added with a wink that warmed me and wounded me at once.

I had no one special to bring.

I hesitated about going alone, but I went.

As I waited for the music to begin, an announcement crackled through the auditorium:

"Maestro will not be conducting tonight. He was taken ill. His replacement is Marcus," the voice finished, but the name barely registered.

My heart sank. “He fevered,” I said to no one in particular.

The orchestra began. I sat, straining to stay present. But eventually, the music reached me. It threaded its way into my chest, loosening the knot of disappointment. Gustavo wasn’t there, but the music still carried him.

POINTY BOOTS

It was a Saturday night, and all I wanted was to curl up on the couch with Rocky tucked against my legs. Shan texted: "Did you go on that date?"

I called her.

She picked up, laughing. "You didn't go, huh?"

"I didn't tell you? I called him last night to firm up the plans —but really, it was to hear his voice."

"And?"

"It was squeaky. Like, helium squeaky. I canceled."

"Oh no," she groaned. "Everything else seemed great."

"It did."

She laughed again. "Well, I'm still texting with Tom. Two months now, and I can't get him to meet."

"So odd," I exhaled. "It's exhausting."

"Almost not worth it," she said. "I did meet the hockey player. He looked nothing like his pictures. They were definitely someone else in those pictures. And I don't think he actually ever played hockey. He just watches it on TV."

"What the heck! Did you stay?"

"Not long. I told him I needed to go to sleep."

We laughed hard, the kind of sisterly laugh only we find funny.

I paused. "What kind of shoes did he wear?"

We had an ongoing philosophy: You can tell a lot about a guy by the car he drives and the shoes he wears. I preferred Jeeps and Olukais.

Shan chuckled. "Pointy."

We laughed again—sharp and strangely comforting.

BENEATH OUR ANSWERS

As the weeks turned to months, my life in D.C. narrowed to two paths: the hospital and the trails. The city's energy felt distant, like I was just observing it from the edges. But in the woods, Rocky and I found refuge, where silence let my thoughts untangle and nature restored me.

At work, I settled in. My coworkers, once reserved, slowly warmed up, offering tips on IV technique and outpatient rhythm. The connections weren't deep, but they were enough. Outside of work, I stopped dating. I just needed a break.

At Sibley, we treated various cancers, including gastrointestinal, sarcoma, and breast cancers. Breast cancer seemed to strike younger and younger, rewriting lives before they had fully begun.

Laura was one of them. Diagnosed at just 27, her story unfolded with both courage and heartbreak. Laura stood out immediately—effervescent, warm, impossible to miss. Her brunette wig styled with a movie-star elegance that brought a radiant energy to the infusion room. She wasn't always my patient, but her warmth pulled people in.

"Hey, Laura, how are you feeling today?"

"Great, thank you, Tara."

As I accessed her mediport, she chatted about her husband's weekly commutes to New York. Laura was usually alone. Her mother had passed away from cancer years earlier, and her father drifted in only once in a while.

"How was your weekend?" she asked.

"I hiked with my dog," I said, thinking about my uneventful weekend. "How about yours?"

"Good." She hesitated.

I waited, hoping she'd say more, but her voice had changed—quieter, distant. "Do you have kids?" I asked, immediately regretting it. I wished I'd asked something gentler, something that didn't ask her to reopen a wound.

"No." Her eyes filled. "I had my ovaries removed a couple of years ago."

"I'm so sorry, Laura." My face flushed with regret—for missing her history and for asking a question I dreaded myself. "That was inconsiderate of me."

Her voice wasn't sharp, but it carried an edge. "It's okay. I'll probably never be over it, but my dog helps." She tried to smile, and it almost held.

"Dogs are great," I offered, but she was no longer interested in my small talk.

Before I left my travel position, I said goodbye to Laura. She stood, arms open, pulling me into a tight embrace, the kind that made everything feel forgiven.

"Enjoy whatever you do until the next time I see you," she said, warm but weighted.

"Likewise, Laura." I wanted to believe we'd meet again, but I wasn't sure.

Laura changed the way I listened. She taught me to pause, to consider what someone might carry beneath their answers. I wish I'd asked about her passions, and about her mother, who shaped her in ways I only glimpsed.

Now I let conversations unfold at their own pace. I resist filling the silence with words. Because sometimes, in the silence is where we hear.

VITALS IN MOTION

Heidi was one of the best parts of Sibley Cancer Center.

She was supposed to be retiring, but scaled back to part-time instead. Somehow, she was there most days with me. If they asked her to pick up a shift, she couldn't say no.

Lucky for me—Heidi made me laugh all day.

One afternoon, she was working with a "VIP" patient. Stiff, pressed, hard to read. She wrapped the blood pressure cuff around his arm, took his vitals, and walked away.

With the machine still attached.

The cuff tugged, and I heard him yelp from a few chairs down. Heidi turned around like she'd just stolen something. She held it together long enough to apologize and uncuff him.

But I didn't.

I was halfway into my church laughter.

Heidi always found the crack in a moment, the place where a laugh could slip in, even in a room that wasn't asking for it.

REARVIEW

In the quiet of the dark morning, I drove east. I glanced at D.C. in my rearview mirror, still looking back. The city shimmered in early light, as if morning had slipped the switch from dark to day. If only I could flip something in myself, make wanderlust optional, restlessness quiet.

My Altima was stuffed to the brim with my life. Rocky claimed the passenger seat the moment I started packing, his posture upright, eyes alert, determined not to be left behind. Rescue dogs carry that kind of memory. I reached over and patted his back.

"It's always *we*, buddy. New York, here we come."

The kaleidoscope of warm hues transformed the skyline. Summer was coming, and the earth was ready for it. We drove east without many goodbyes. My coworkers were kind, but other than Heidi, they were temporary. That's the rhythm of travel nursing: try a place, stay if it fits. I'd extended once, but when they asked again, I said no. I was lonely in D.C., and the idea of a city that never sleeps, near family, felt like a hopeful antidote.

My phone rang.

I smiled before I even answered. "Maya!"

"Well, hello, Tara!"

We'd emailed now and then, but this was our first real phone conversation.

"NYC, huh?"

It was so good to hear her voice. "Yes! Memorial Sloan Kettering." I sounded far too excited about a cancer center to a cancer patient. "How are you?" My words felt heavy.

"I skied this winter," she said, and I could tell she knew that would make me smile. "Being out on a mountain again felt *amazing*!"

"That's incredible, Maya!" My eyes welled up. "What kind of day was it?"

"Bluebird." Her voice was strong, and I could hear her smiling.

"I'm all smiles," I told her, wiping my tears.

"I knew you'd want to hear that. I'm heading out for a hike today," she added. "Thought of you; you still owe me one."

"Ah, I know . . ." I sighed. "Soak it all in."

"I do. Every day."

We laughed like we'd summited something.

It was bittersweet. I wanted to be there, on the trails beside her. We used to talk about it like it could actually happen. I could've made a long detour, found a way to see her. Life got in the way—the way it always does when we think we have all the time. But even unkept promises have their own kind of grace. She made it out. She was *living*.

The sun climbed higher, brushing the sky gold. The darkness was gone, the light taking over. I thought about all the small moments in a day when this shift happens. All life's beauty passing through when we aren't paying attention.

PART III

2014—NEW YORK, NY

MEMORIAL SLOAN KETTERING

THE ONE THAT GOT AWAY

Memorial Sloan Kettering was the one that got away.

From the moment I stepped inside, with cucumber-filled glass water jugs and window walls spilling natural light, something in me aligned—a feeling I hadn't realized I'd been missing.

I'd started my travel nurse assignment at Memorial Sloan Kettering (MSK), and orientation began at the main campus. As I walked the corridor, something in me steadied. Lining the hallways were photographs of oceans and mountaintops, images that spoke to my nature-loving soul. Soft piano music floated through the air, dulling the chaos of my commute. Orientation was draining, but MSK made it feel lighter.

The hospital chaplain took the stage.

Her full black robe cloaked her small frame, only white hair visible behind the podium. She dragged a stool over and adjusted the microphone. "Good morning. I am Sister Agnes." Her voice was shaky, but her tone sincere. A chaplain? I'd been bracing for a firehose of logistics and policy. Silently, I tucked my flip phone into my bag.

"I'm here to tell you one important thing," she said, scanning the crowd. "But I need all eyes and ears on me," she added, raising an eyebrow. The crowd stilled. Phones vanished into bags.

"That's better," she said with a grin, earning a soft ripple of laughter.

"I won't be discussing IV skills or insurance policies. Instead, let us talk about the souls you'll heal." She had a Santa Claus quality to her, ancient, disarming, full of wonder. "Let me tell you a tale."

And she did—story after story. The patients' voices came through her, though the details were hers. It became clear she made her presence felt by listening, not with protocol, but with her heart.

Before stepping away, Sister Agnes gave a parting message that rooted itself deep within me:

"There is more to healing than medicine.

There is healing in human connection.

Don't get caught in the rat race of nursing.

Don't just hear each other..."

She paused, then offered a lesson that would shape everything that came after: "Listen. Become a first-class listener."

53RD AND LEXINGTON

Everything at MSK felt like stepping into another world. I worked at the Rockefeller outpatient pavilion on 53rd and Lexington, another towering structure of modern architecture and sleek design.

In the lobby, I was greeted by Nate. Like Oprah, famous without a last name. He radiated charm, with a deep love for people and a booming voice that woke the soul each shift.

"Good morning, Miss Tara," he'd call out, walking around his station, hand extended, smile like the sunrise. That daily moment brought lift—a tiny spark that carried into the rest of the day.

The ninth-floor thoracic oncology unit was equally impressive. Tucked between skyscrapers in midtown Manhattan, it somehow burst with natural light. The waiting room carried the same polished feel—warm-toned walls, fresh fruit-water jugs, and nature prints. My coworkers greeted me with easy smiles and open arms.

If I needed a hand with an IV, I could ask anyone. They made me laugh till I cried—the kind that made patients peek out of curtains asking if we were all right. We were wildly different, like dogs of every breed, but we worked as one.

Conversations were candid, pure New York City, late-night, straight-talk energy. I admired their candor. There was no pretense. Just grab your chart and flow. The place ran like a well-oiled machine, humming with purpose and camaraderie.

THORACIC 9

Thoracic 9 treated various lung cancers, mesothelioma, small-cell lung cancer (SCLC), non-small-cell lung cancer (NSCLC), thymoma, and mediastinal tumors. Across from the treatment rooms sat the thoracic doctors and their collaborative team, always accessible, never distant. Chairside during reactions, quick with a hand, steady with an answer. No question was too small.

Some patients had smoking histories, some chemical exposures. Others were mystery diagnoses, with no clear origin, just cells blooming where they shouldn't, lungs bearing a story no one could trace.

The morning I met Nancy, we were down a nurse. Everything felt one beat behind. Patient charts lined the station, and we grabbed one, did our checks, then told the Session Assistant, our ship's captain, that we were ready. They managed everything: schedules, drug follow-ups with pharmacy, patient flow. I grabbed Nancy's chart. New diagnosis: small-cell lung cancer (SCLC). Fast-moving, aggressive.

I walked into her room, and the smell of cigarettes wrapped

around me like a second skin. It was dense, familiar, part of the air, part of her.

"Hello," Nancy said. Her deep, raspy voice reverberated off the walls. "You must be Tara." Her eyes sparkled with warmth and mischief.

"I am. And you must be Nancy."

"You got it," she grinned, then gestured to her husband. "This is Ted."

Ted looked like a polished lawyer—slicked-back hair, tailored clothes, charm that came standard. I shook his hand, noted the nice smile. But beneath it, I saw fear. I wished I could reassure him. Instead, I launched into the treatment plan.

"The chemotherapy attacks the rapidly dividing cells," I began. "Which are your good cells, too, so there are some side effects—"

Nancy cut me off. "I don't want to know any of those, Tara. Please. Tell me about yourself."

I'd learned over the years that patients often held on to the nurse who helped them through their first hard day. Nancy was already holding on to me.

I folded the education paperwork and slid it to Ted. We'd talk later.

"I just closed on a condo," I offered, reaching for a cheerful fact. My life felt rather vanilla.

Nancy lit up. Ted smiled, too, nudging the drug sheet aside. He already knew she wasn't interested.

"That's so exciting!" Nancy leaned forward, genuinely curious. "Tell me more."

"About the chemo or about my condo?"

Nancy cackled, a sound that turned immediately into a cough.

"Our son's about your age. If you're single, that is . . ."

I nodded. "I am." Always awkward, especially here.

She grinned, delighted. "So, what do you like to do for fun?"

I stood, easing us back toward the work. "I like to hike. But I do have to get your medicine going. Can I get you anything? Something to eat or drink?"

"Nope. Though I could really use a smoke," Nancy joked. "To stay calm."

"Points for honesty," I said, smiling. Nancy wasn't one for pretense.

Throughout the day, she kept checking in on me—my condo, my schedule, the small details of my life she'd pulled out earlier.

"What's your favorite thing to do?" she asked. Her curiosity was disarming.

"I like skiing," I said, instantly transported to the mountains.

"Oh! My son snowboards too." A wink.

I exhaled, half-laughing.

"How about we go over the possible side effects now? I can grab you a drink or a snack first if you want."

"All this waiting on me, the blankets, the bed…if I ignore the poison, it's almost spa-like," she chuckled.

"We try to make you comfortable," I offered gently.

"I could get used to this," she said. "Feels, well…kind of like Stockholm Syndrome." She chuckled.

I laughed. It was funny because it was true how treatment routines settle into strange comfort, how we adapt.

Her chuckle cracked into a jagged cough, the kind that rattles a room. She tried to smile through it, but the cough broke it apart.

THE FLOOR THAT HELD US

Thoracic 9 had its own rhythm. Some days were so heavy, we didn't look at each other until the shift was over. Other days, we laughed so hard I worried my mascara would run into the anti-nausea meds waiting on the counter. It was the kind of unit that shouldn't have worked—too many personalities, too much chaos—but it did. Because of the people.

Raya and Selene were the undisputed queens of locker room storytelling. No filters, no warnings. Their stories were plentiful. Loud ones. Juli, our IV whisperer and steady center of gravity, would just chuckle and shake her head while threading a 22-gauge IV like she was lacing a shoe. Tony, the medical assistant, was our in-house pot-stirrer. He'd drop a single suggestive question into the conversation like a lit match and stroll out of the room, only to return five minutes later like he had no idea why we were still debating.

Kenz was spirited, always two tasks behind. Her flustered state entertained us more than we ever admitted. Anne ran at an even higher frequency, more frenetic, like a hummingbird trying to document a tornado—chaotic, yes, but impossible not to love.

Kylie, a quick-witted brunette with an impeccable delivery, a rare blend of lawyer turned nurse, had a knack for turning even the most humdrum situation into something laughable. Her one-liners hit like darts, and somehow, she always knew exactly what I was going through before I had the words for it. She didn't say much, but when she did, it usually rearranged the air in the room.

And then there was Laura and Kate. Calm, kind, unshakably decent. The kind of nurses who made you want to try harder just by standing next to them.

We had our own choreography: who to go to when a port stopped flushing, who had the best dating story, who could make you laugh mid-storm. It wasn't always graceful, but we *worked*. And in between blood draws and emergencies, we found something like family.

I didn't know what kind of nurse I'd become when I started Thoracic 9.

Turns out, it's the people who shape the nurse.

TAOS OR BIG SKY

"Is Raya here today?" Maureen's voice trembled.

"No, she is not. I'm Tara, though, and I would love to be your nurse today," I said, hoping for a calming effect.

Maureen offered a tentative smile. "Okay, Tara, I'd like that." She paused. "It's just Raya always gets my IV." IV anxiety was common, and patients grew attached to their nurses' IV skills.

"Well, I am pretty good myself," I said, trying to sound confident.

"You better be," a strong voice interrupted. Ed barreled through the curtain. "I'm Ed, Maureen's husband." With his white hair pushed back and collared confidence, Ed looked like a retired CEO ready to play some golf. Maureen shook her head, a mixture of exasperation and affection in her eyes.

"All set," I said, securing the catheter.

"Wow, I did not even feel that," Maureen sighed in relief. "Well, the worst part is over. Now we can chat."

I wished there was time to chat, but I needed to be on the other side of the curtain. Patients often turned small moments into personal exchanges because connection had its own urgency. Maybe they understood the fleeting better than most, how much a minute could offer.

"So, where are you from, Tara?" Maureen asked. Before I could answer, she leaned in a little, her questions picking up pace. "Are you married? Any children?"

I chuckled. "Not married, no children, and I live in New Jersey with my dog."

"What's a girl like you doing living alone?" Ed's tone was a mix of teasing and concern.

"I don't live alone, Ed—I live with my dog," I volleyed back. "What about you two? How long have you been married?"

Years of love and history passed between them. They'd dated from their late teens to early twenties. Maureen wanted to get married, but Ed needed more time. They broke up, only to be reunited by fate. Back then, people drifted for real—no social media, no easy way to find someone again.

"It was pouring — one of those sideways rains," Ed started.

"The kind where you look at your feet to keep the rain from hitting your eyes," Maureen's voice softened. "I was 39; it had been 13 years—"

"—she walked right into me, umbrella and all," Ed cut in, his expression nostalgic.

A ripple of goosebumps rose on my arms.

"I was shocked to see him." Maureen's smile deepened the lines around her eyes.

"It was like a gift from the heavens." Ed raised his arms, smiling. It was the kind of smile that made me forget how intense he'd been moments earlier.

"We were married within the year," Maureen continued. "Kids didn't happen for us, though." Her face shifted. "We missed the boat on that."

Ed pivoted in his chair. "So, we traveled a lot. We skied in the winters and sailed in the summers."

"That's a beautiful story," I said, moved. "And I love skiing!"

"Oh yeah?" Ed stood, eager to engage. "Where do you go—out West, I hope?"

"Vermont, mostly, but I've been to Colorado," I said, already half-turned toward the curtain. Ed perked up, talking faster now.

"Okay, so this season, go to Taos, New Mexico or Big Sky, Montana," he said, launching into a passionate sales pitch that had nothing to do with cancer and everything to do with wonder.

I hadn't planned a ski trip. But as they shared more of their journeys, I began to wonder why not.

TUSCANY

I crowdsourced. I asked my sister and texted my friends. Most were too busy working to go on an impromptu ski trip, but Callie was interested. She was still working at Wilmot Cancer Center, and three 12s a week left space for spontaneity.

"Any interest in a ski trip out West the week of February 22nd?" I texted. The dates weren't flexible. I was just about to shift from travel nurse to a full-time position at MSK.

"Yes!" she replied immediately. Callie rarely said no—to last-minute trips, to night shifts, to life.

"A patient suggested Taos or Big Sky," I added. I was indecisive.

"Montana," she texted back. "I always wanted to go there!"

"Perfect. Big Sky it is." I smiled to myself.

My phone rang.

"Hey." Just one word, but her tone dropped, and I knew.

"What's up?"

"Benny passed." I heard the exhale, like she'd been holding her breath since the moment she learned. The shift was so abrupt it felt like someone had yanked the cord on the moment. A pang of sadness moved through me. My heart ached. I had looked up his restaurant during my last visit. I hadn't gone. I could still see him lifting one eyebrow when he was about to challenge me.

"Everyone wanted to tell you. I think they were waiting for you to ask." I'd left the cancer center a year and a half earlier. When you leave a place like that, you don't expect updates. You don't expect to hear who passed. But the stories keep unfolding, even when you're no longer there to witness them.

"Did you see him?" I asked. I wanted to know the man he was at the end.

"He wasn't here," she said. "He was in Italy. His wife stopped by to tell us."

There was a warmth in her voice, like she was remembering something she thought I needed to hear.

"Living life," I said with an exhale. Not to her. To Benny.

Benny was in Tuscany when he relapsed. It was within three years of his initial diagnosis. He sold his business and rented a place with his wife. His family trickled in for however long they could stay. He spent his last days fishing, enjoying his freshly caught cuisine and the love surrounding him.

"Thanks for telling me," I said, picturing him, remembering his sharp humor, his angry wisdom.

"So…Big Sky?"

"Big Sky it is."

FEEL THAT FIRE

I wasn't Nancy's nurse that day, but I stopped by to check in. On a ten-room floor, you always knew when the patients you needed to see were there.

"Here," she said, extending a long, gift-wrapped rectangle. "I picked up something for your new condo." I smiled, caught off guard. I hadn't realized we'd crossed into friendship. It snuck up on me, like most real things do. Inside the paper was a wooden sign. It read: *Welcome.* Simple. Thoughtful. My eyes welled.

"I thought you could use a little decoration," she said. "With your schedule, it's probably hard to get to those finishing touches."

"It's perfect," I said softly. "Thank you, Nancy."

"So…any new men in your life?" she asked, sounding like my mother.

"Nope. No news on that front." I laughed, casually dismissing my singlehood.

"Oh, you'll meet someone. You can't hurry love." Her tone softened into something wise.

"Yeah, honestly, nothing's felt right yet." It was only our second encounter, but her presence felt instantly familiar—that unplaceable sense that you've known someone longer than you have.

"You'll know when it feels right." Nancy smiled.

"I've heard that before. I've definitely mastered the doesn't-feel-right part," I joked.

She laughed, her wonderful laugh. "I did too. I didn't get married until I was 38."

She paused, eyes steady. "It's fire. You need to feel that fire." Then, softer still, "Hopefully I'm here to hear about him."

The words hung in the air, fragile. For a moment, neither of us filled the silence.

"Me too," I said. Nancy gave me a wink. I half-smiled back.

At the desk, I set down her wooden sign, still carrying the weight of her presence. Some people stay with you.

FIND MY RUN

"Is Tara here today?" Maureen's voice drifted through the curtain, sweet but certain.

"She is," Kylie replied. "But I grabbed your chart. Can I take care of you today?"

At MSK, patients often requested nurses. It was part of the culture; attachments formed fast, and satisfaction mattered. But the expectation was to show up fully before passing the baton. Try to earn the connection. Every patient deserved our best, and that's what we tried to give.

"Oh, I'm sure you're great," Maureen said, but her tone wavered, like the words didn't quite match the feeling behind them.

I stepped around the curtain. "Good morning!"

Ed's face lit up.

"You two gave me the push," I said without pause, "Big Sky is officially booked for February." I felt my heart flutter with excitement.

Ed reached into his back pocket and unfolded a trail map, edges still crisp as if it had never been opened.

"Big Sky, Montana," I read aloud. I exhaled, caught off guard by how much this trip already meant. "You brought this for me?" I asked, voice softening under the weight of the gesture. Like he couldn't wait for me to see it for myself.

Ed nodded. I smiled and held out my arms. We met in an awkward hug, his jacket stiff against my cheek and smelling faintly of aftershave a decade out of style.

"This trail," he said, unfolding the map, "Maur would take off ahead of me, leaving me in the dust. It was a black, beautiful glades, but steep." His eyes went wide, as if remembering just how steep it really was.

I raised an eyebrow. "So, you're the black diamond type?"

Maureen waved a hand, amused. "I just loved being in those glades." Her smile turned meditative. Her eyes closed, and I could almost see it too. "Between the trees. It was peaceful. Empty. All I could hear," she whispered, "was my breath. My heart. And the snow falling." She opened her eyes. I wanted that moment to be real again for her.

The Alaris pump beeped.

Her expression shifted, like she'd woken up in the wrong world.

"Thank you both," I said, leaning in to hug her, this one easy, mutual.

"Hey, maybe you'll find yourself a nice man," Maureen smiled.

I smirked, polite and practiced. I'd heard it before. One couple insisted I'd meet my future husband at the mall on Christmas Eve. I did not go to the mall. And I was still single.

"You'll find my run," she added with a knowing smile.

I slipped the trail map into my back pocket, thinking about the unlikely trio we'd become.

BIG SKY

Big Sky country got its name for good reason.

The endless skies stretched uninterrupted to the horizon, like Earth's roof compared to the NYC blacktop. The wildland mirrored the sky above as our shuttle bus wove up the mountains, tracing the river that ran through them.

The driver didn't seem to brake. Snow lined the pavement and piled on the windshield as his wipers thrashed in overdrive. My jaw tightened. I gripped my hands in prayer.

His knuckles weren't white. Mine definitely were.

I exhaled as the shuttle came to a screeching stop at my slopeside lodge. Years of patient inspiration rationalized this splurge. Callie was scheduled to arrive around midnight. Hopefully with a different driver; otherwise, I wondered if I'd end up flying solo.

I stepped into my home for the next five days. It was a log cabin lodge, rustic in the way mountain places are—warm wood, heavy beams, quiet corners. Elk and moose fixtures lined the lobby, and old skis had been repurposed as wall art. Beyond the entry was an open space with a 30-foot-high ceiling. Mountains filled with massive pines that stopped long before the jagged ridges and snowcapped summits. My inner child did backflips as I looked up in awe at the rugged peaks I'd soon explore.

My stomach growled, reminding me of the unintended fast I wanted to break. The man sitting next to me on the airplane had given me a restaurant suggestion. For most of our flight to Bozeman, he spat out Big Sky facts. I tuned out much of his gibberish, but my hungry mind held on to the good eats.

I brought my journal and trail map along and took the 10-minute stroll to the restaurant. I was breathy; the air felt thin but clean. The snow was high and fresh. Kids climbed a snow pile's peaks and slid down on their butts and bellies, making high-pitched squeals. Parents sat on the Adirondack chairs designed from vintage skis, sipping après beverages and laughing. A group of teenagers congregated around the outdoor fireplace. I lowered my sunglasses from my forehead; even the setting sun through the clouds felt bright.

I stepped into the restaurant, the snow-bright world going dark as my eyes adjusted. Being single and alone, I made a beeline for the bar, passing the coupled patrons in fancy attire. It stung a bit. Not sharp, not surprising. Just familiar.

At 33, I'd gotten used to walking into places alone. Still, moments like this had a way of reminding me. Wine bottles lined the back of the bar. I slid onto a stool in the far corner and ordered a glass of wine and a salad to start.

I broke my fast with a sip of red wine, tasting every bit of it. The aroma of Italian spices made my stomach sing some more. I opened my journal and set aside my bookmark—Ed's trail map. A group of men took over the barstools beside me. I smiled out of friendliness and turned back to my journal. I wrote about Darren. The solitude sent me straight into familiar questions: Did I jump ship too soon? Does something more really exist?

"Is that salad good?" the man beside me asked. He had sharp eyes and dusky brown hair.

"So good," I answered, keeping it brief. But my smile kept the small talk alive. I quickly learned this man's wife was also an oncology nurse, and the conversation carried with the coincidence. I enjoyed chatting with strangers; it was far better to be in the moment than in my head. His friends lining the bar chimed in, buying me another glass of wine and small-talking it up. Within minutes, the one with the voice I couldn't place—deep, accented, and oddly familiar—gravitated toward me, drawn to my trail map like it held answers.

He wore his flannel cuffs rolled back, revealing muscular, hairy forearms as he leaned into the map. Pointing from one run to the next, he methodically described the chairlifts and suitable terrain. I was more drawn to his voice—warm, deliberate—than the ins and outs of Big Sky Montana. With salt-and-pepper hair and an intellectual's glasses, his age was mysterious.

"Dave," he said, offering up his hand and a charming smile.

Cupping his strong hand with mine, everything else faded away — the chatter, the music, all of it.

"Tara," I said, smiling for too long.

His hazel eyes held my gaze. Heat rushed from my heart to my cheeks. My mind went blank. I was left in whatever that moment was. It felt different than before—no tightened jaw, no polite deflection. Just a warm hand in mine, and the strange calm of letting it be what it was.

"Maybe we'll cross paths on the mountain," Dave said, his deep octave hitting me in a way I didn't expect, as his friends gestured it was time to head out. Holding up to their higher standards, the restaurant only allowed pizza to be taken out. I waved my goodbyes and was left alone again.

I closed my journal, pages heavy with failed relationships,

and trekked into the fresh snow. I didn't yet know how the place worked—the vast mountain above, the quaintness of the base area below—or that Dave and I would keep finding each other in the days ahead, at a bar, on chairlifts, in conversations that felt like the start of something.

ROOTING FOR EACH OTHER

The unit buzzed as always, call bells ringing, voices half-raised. I'd barely dropped my coat before Ed chimed in.

"So, what did you think?" Ed called out.

"And did you meet a nice man?" Maureen's voice sounded weaker, and her clothing looked looser. Her smile was still there, but it didn't reach her eyes the way it used to.

It was my first day back from Big Sky, still buzzing with fresh air, adrenaline, and something like possibility.

Ed stared through me, waiting.

"I loved the mountain, Ed."

He whipped another trail map from his back pocket.

"Show me where you went," he said—gruff and somehow friendly at the same time.

I smiled. Of course he had a trail map.

"Well?" Maureen's interest was not on the trail map.

"I did, Maureen."

Her smile widened.

"I like him, but he lives in Pittsburgh." My smile widened too.

Ed creased the map into its pristine fold. "Oh, come on. Is

that your only excuse?" He leaned in, suddenly invested. "You can't travel?"

"Well, we're planning a trip to Stowe."

Ed's tone shifted—protective beneath the bark. "Oh, this is moving fast. Tell me more about this guy."

A call bell rang next to me.

"Well, he liked your trail map."

Ed's grimace softened.

"You have to promise me one thing."

I could only imagine.

"Oh, Ed, what now?" Maureen's eyes lifted in a tired roll.

I braced for something sarcastic. Ed had an arsenal.

"We want a wedding invitation."

Maureen and I laughed.

Ed persisted, poker-faced. "I am serious."

"If I ever get married, Ed, it's a deal." I never wanted a wedding, but Ed and I shook on it anyway. His hand was warm, mine reluctant. In that pause, we sealed something that mattered. It wasn't the wedding that made me smile—it was the way people root for each other.

SELENE

Dave and I departed Big Sky with a feeling of words left unsaid. On my flight home, as I stared off into the vastness of the sky, I wondered if we'd cross paths again. I'd made friends on vacation before, when reality fades and time bends. The goodbyes stay open-ended, and the moment dissolves on landing. As the plane touched down, a bittersweet melancholy settled in, the quiet ache of what could have been.

The next day, Dave texted me a picture of his racquetball game. Odd, but welcome. Our texts turned into phone calls, then plans for a ski trip before winter slipped into spring. We settled on Stowe, Vermont; he would swing by New Jersey from Pittsburgh to pick me up. Our first date.

"You're getting your own room, right?" Selene, my coworker —the very cerebral queen of sex conversation—asked. She didn't look up from her screen, her words crisp, as if issuing a professional decree. I swiveled in my chair.

"You think I should?" I wasn't planning on it. Selene gave a heavy, affirmative nod—almost bobblehead in its certainty.

"I would. Even if you like this guy, it'd be better for the first trip." Selene exuded confidence all the time; even her strut looked purposeful. She spoke like someone who rarely second-guessed herself, a woman who made decisions swiftly and expected others to keep up.

"I always get my own room for situations like this," she stated, unfazed.

I paused, unsure how to respond. This situation felt unique. "You're in this pickle often?"

Her chuckle was my answer. "Get yourself a room, Duff." She always called me Duff, which I liked; my teammates gave me that nickname, and something about her carried that same teammate energy.

I glanced at my phone and saw a message notification from Dave.

"Is a king bed okay?" Accompanied by the nonchalance of the sunglasses emoji, I showed Selene. She smiled.

'Hey, I don't care if you marry this dude; it's your first date."

I wrote Dave back: "Sounds good."

Sometimes, the heart just knows.

STOWE

Dusk settled, the sky streaked in amber and violet. I breathed deeply as Dave's Jeep Cherokee pulled into my parking lot. I felt a small lift in my chest. Will I still like this guy, or will it be like those online dates, so different from the jigsaw stories I assembled in my head? My palms sweated and my heart skipped. Should I trust my instincts?

Dave stepped out of the truck, his walk suggesting his left leg was heavier than the right. I noticed the way people carry things—in their posture, their pace, their silence.

He flashed his charming smile. My stomach dipped.

Heat rushed through my veins, a quick surge that met my nerves head-on. My lungs finally let go. He reached for my bags, his flannel rolled at the cuff. "I got the bags," he said coolly. His deep voice—touched with that soft Pittsburgh edge he swore he didn't have—was all I heard. The stories in my head dissipated. The world slowed.

On the drive to Stowe, I felt at ease. We talked, we laughed; there was no hurry. He felt familiar, like someone I'd known all my life and suddenly wanted to know everything about.

Ten hours into Dave's drive from Pittsburgh, his hand

started to cramp. "Here, let me see—I'll massage it." I took his hand, working my thumb into his palm. His hazel eyes squinted with a smile. For a moment, everything else fell away.

Massive snow piles surrounded the hotel. Its timeless magic awakened something in me. Inside, Dave poured me a glass of red wine. We sat on the couch, conversation flowing as easily as it had in the car. He smiled at me—the same smile from the day we met, the one that communicated more than an interest in my trail map. He reached for my hand. His touch was electric, sending ripples through my veins. My heart galloped. I leaned in. Something tipped from friendship into something else. I felt the gravity shift, the sensation of the fall.

The feeling was fire.

HOLDING BOTH

There's always a moment after a vacation when I forget I'm supposed to numb people's veins with poison.

On the commute in, I felt like I was still in the mountains. I smiled at the sunrise like someone who hasn't seen 8 a.m. with fluorescent lights in a while. My gait was looser, my skin smelled faintly of firewood and fresh snow. I drank my coffee slow.

But then the unit door opened. And I remembered.

The clatter of call bells, the beep of infusion pumps, the scent of hand sanitizer and warmed blankets rushed in before my badge even scanned. Within minutes, I was setting up chemotherapy, reviewing labs, checking for neutropenia, verifying med doses.

The nurse part of me snapped in.

And yet, under the scrub top, something felt different.

Maybe it's the memory of defeated eyes before we hugged for the last time.

Maybe it's the ghost of the lodge fire still warming my bones.

Maybe it's the man who held my hand across two states and made everything feel easier.

Or maybe it's all of it—how being an oncology nurse means holding love and loss at once.

Some days, I think I'm getting better at it.

Other days, I feel like I'm learning to walk again, with two different kinds of gravity.

WITH A HEART UNTAMED

I approached the nurses' station just as Hank strolled into the infusion center. He wore the same worn-out yellow ball cap he always did, gripping the hefty Normandy book I never saw him without. He looked like he was about to make me laugh all afternoon.

"I'll take Hank today," I told the charge nurse.

It was the first time I claimed a patient. The words felt strange, but Hank was already grinning.

"Did you just pick me?" His smile stretched wide as he pointed to his chest.

"I sure did, Hank. I'm due for some laughs."

"Oh, the pressure's on—what's my status on your funny list anyway?" he asked, still smiling.

"Oh, you're up there, Hank—number three. Just something to keep you working for," I said with a smirk.

Hank's shoulders lifted with pride as he placed his book on his lap.

"Same spot as last week," he said, pointing to his bookmark. We chuckled.

"You need a new book."

It was my perfect segue to ask if he'd ever look at my writing. But if I asked Hank, it would take us beyond patient and nurse—into something deeper. Something I wasn't sure I was ready for.

We both started at once.

"So, my b—"

"I was thinking—"

He shifted in his seat. "Go ahead."

"No, you first," I said, my confidence wavering.

"So, I was thinking of taking my wife to Arizona," Hank continued. "She can play tennis, and I can golf all day. All the meals included. And it'll be warm."

"Sounds like your heaven."

Hank nodded, raising an eyebrow. "Well…let's not rule that destination out either," he chuckled. I couldn't help but laugh along with him.

He placed his book aside and rolled up his sleeves, ready to tell more stories. We talked about his recent visit to his son's, his Thanksgiving plans, and the family trip they had coming up for Christmas—stories that made my ribs ache from laughter.

"All set," I said, deaccessing his mediport.

"I'm done? Just like that?"

"Just like that."

Hank always lingered on his exit. Likely because he wanted to get in one more joke or story. And he always did.

"I'd like to go golf now, but I don't know if I want to deal with 'the people,' you know?" He smiled, wry.

"Wear your headphones," I joked. He once told me he wore his headphones floating under his shirt—unplugged, disconnected—so he wouldn't have to talk to "the people."

"People love the superficials," he mused. "They love to ask, 'What do you do for work?' And it's not because they want to know what I do—it's because they want to tell me what they do."

He stood, anchoring himself. "And they want to tell me all about it." His hands gestured, miming these fictitious people unloading their life stories onto him. "Who cares." He waved, as if the hypothetical crowd were beside him.

I smiled in amusement. Small talk dressed up as connection, everyone waiting for their turn to speak.

As Hank lingered, my book maintained its quiet persistence. Should I ask him?

"So, will I see you next time?" Hank asked.

"I hope so, Hank," I said with a smile, carrying the weight of the words left unspoken.

"Even a sick old man likes being picked."

I shook my head, smiling.

He hesitated, just for a second.

"All right, well—hey. I'll be in touch."

His tried-and-true exit line.

He peeled himself away.

Hank didn't like goodbyes either.

Maybe that's why he lingered.

They felt so final, sometimes.

STILL HER

The email came on a Tuesday.

I was hunched at the nurses' station, clicking through labs and half a yogurt, when her name popped in my inbox like a Post-it from another life.

Behind me, Raya was trying to convince Selene that her boyfriend's silence was not because she was balancing two boyfriends at once. Juli shook her head as she settled into charge for the day. Tony sang, "Today's gonna be a good day," as he walked by in a borrowed doctor's coat and a mischievous grin.

"I took a trip to Vermont this winter. The snow was perfect, and I almost forgot I was ever sick." Maya attached a photo: bundled in a powder-blue parka, goggles perched on her head, the ridgelines of the Green Mountains behind her like something hand-painted. She looked flushed, happy, real.

"I had a full year of teaching kindergarten again. I wouldn't trade them. Well, most days."

I smiled, relieved. She still had that dry, untouchable wit.

Nearly a year out from transplant—teaching, hiking, skiing, living.

"I've been having these little blips. Forgot what day it was. Misplaced my phone in the refrigerator. I figured it was just chemo brain, but my oncologist ordered a scan just in case."

I reread that paragraph twice, unsure whether to laugh or worry. With Maya, it was always a little of both.

"Vertical. Still stubborn. You owe me a picture. I'm sure you're heading somewhere amazing."

The unit didn't pause for my nostalgia.

Behind me, someone was swearing about a missing drug. Kenz rushed by holding three charts and her breath. Anne shouted, "We're out of rooms!" like the place might burst into flames. Kylie was giggling behind her, and I couldn't help but laugh along.

I wrote Maya back between pre-meds. I asked her how Vermont felt, hoping she'd give me the kind of answer only she could—the kind that made ordinary days feel extraordinary.

And just like that, she was back in my world. Moving forward, hopeful. Still her.

EVEREST

Madeline was the kind of wild that made me feel boring.

"I climbed Mt. Everest," she said, beaming, scrolling through photos on her phone. "I was being treated for cancer," she added, handing me her phone. "My friend called and said, 'I'm climbing Everest—come.' He had everything planned. Still, I deliberated. But then I thought, it's all set up for me. If not now, when?"

She raised her eyes to meet mine, brimming with pride.

Madeline was in her 40s, wearing Birkenstocks and a halo of messy dark curls, youth still woven into her style in a way that felt effortless. She looked like she should be drinking tea by a wood stove in Vermont. Instead, she sat in a hospital recliner, wearing a port and a smile like she knew something the rest of us didn't.

I knew very little about her prognosis, treatment, or timeline. It was a simple visit—just a port flush and labs. Sometimes, I preferred the mystery. The kind that felt full of possibility.

"That's amazing," I said, swiping through stunning Himalayan landscapes.

"I had just gotten the kiss of death," she said. "I didn't know how long I had. And still...I deliberated."

"You had every reason to hesitate," I offered.

"Exactly what gave me the push."

I flushed her port with heparin and slid on a Band-Aid.

"I wouldn't have gone without cancer," she admitted. "I think life makes our decisions for us," she said, then paused. "We just have to listen."

I filed that line in my mental cabinet, the kind I'd pull out later when I needed to borrow someone else's courage.

"I would have waited for the 'perfect' time in some far-off future," she said, shaking her head. "You know?"

I did. I was the classic case of Tomorrow.

"So, I spoke to my doctor, she approved it, and I pushed treatment back a week. It all fell into place. I was definitely more fatigued than the rest of the group. But we hired a guide. He carried my pack. I needed breaks. But I did it." Her voice lit up, like the memory sparked something alive in her.

The unit surged behind the curtain, alarms, voices, half-shouted orders. But Madeline held a calm the floor couldn't touch.

"If not now, when, right?" she said, handing me a glossy postcard titled *Himalaya Adventures*. A yoga retreat in India. The invitation looked passed-around, softened and torn at its edges.

She handed it to me like she'd read a page I hadn't written yet.

"Come," she said, like it was that easy.

"Thank you." I stood there, speechless.

"I finally decided I'm going," she added. "I mean, again, here I am, cancer, unknown everything, and I still deliberated."

Sometimes fear is a compass. And sometimes it just holds us in place.

"You like that picture?" she asked, pointing to her phone still in my hand.

"Love it," I said, already hungry for its story.

"That's Kala Patthar," she boomed. "They woke us at 3 a.m. to climb. Unless it was raining, of course. I hoped for rain. You know, we are wired to seek comfort. But no rain," she grinned.

I grinned back, knowing what she meant.

"We climbed and climbed and climbed. I got dizzy. My Sherpa just told me to slow down. We arrived before 5 a.m., and the views were covered in fog. Nothing to see. We were so disappointed." She paused. "I muttered to my friend, 'We paid for this?'" She chuckled. "Typical Americans. Always in a rush to nowhere. The guide said just one word—'Patience.' We stayed. We waited. And then: The clouds parted. Light scattered everywhere—like something from the gods. I couldn't speak. Couldn't move. It was the kind of beauty that makes you forget everything else."

She was still smiling when she looked up. A little breathless, like she was still somewhere on that ridge. "It sure as hell beat my living room."

My smile met hers.

Everest wasn't a trophy. It was a reckoning.

I handed her the yoga invite, but she pushed it into my hand again as she moved to exit.

"No, keep it," she said. "Someday."

I smiled, tucked it into my back pocket, and stepped back into the hum of routine.

WHAT NANCY KNEW

Nancy's son and Ted stood on the other side of the curtain. A look passed between us, speaking the words I didn't want to hear.

"She passed," Ted's voice caught.

I opened my arms and muttered the only words I knew, "I am so sorry, Ted." Ted gripped my shoulders tightly as if I held his last memories of his wife. Through his grip, I felt the rise and fall of his chest. Madeline slipped behind him, pressing her hands into her heart and mouthing a *thank you* as she exited.

"Thank you for everything you do. My mom loved all your conversations," Nancy's son blurted, his voice catching too.

"I loved our conversations," I managed, my voice thick with emotion.

There's a sting in realizing I'll never see someone I'd only just begun to know again. It's part of oncology nursing—the ache and the privilege of it. We all connect better when we feel something real, deep in our bones. And when it's gone, you notice the space it leaves.

Nancy knew something I was only beginning to understand. She knew all that mattered in this life was love—not titles, not accomplishments, not the things we cling to. Nancy reminded me to slow down, not rush love. If we pause and revel in our time with others, we find love all around us.

"Thank you for all you do." Ted released my shoulders and retreated toward the doors. A tug at my heart, a slow exhale.

The yoga invitation stabbed my backside as I slid into my chair. I adjusted it with a smile. There it was again, the pull of possibility against the tug of heartache.

AUGUST 2015

VALLE NEVADO, CHILE

TWO PINK LINES

Madeline told me life makes our decisions if we listen. I was always a sucker for serendipity, but I was still learning how to listen for the big stuff.

My relationship with Dave was still kindling. I loved him—his steadiness, his sense of adventure—and he'd asked me to move to Pittsburgh.

It was only June—we'd met in February—and I wanted more time to let our relationship unfold. I loved my job at MSK, and we had a ski trip planned for August in Chile. I asked him to table the "what are we" conversations until then.

We set out for Chile with the kind of excitement that makes sleep impossible. The flights felt interminable, and the drive from the airport to the mountaintop was one continuous switchback. The driver flew around bends like a roller coaster, and I was car sick by the first turn. But the snowcapped Andes made up for it—bold, rugged peaks reeling us in as we pulled into our home for the week.

As we jumped out of the car, the sun hit our faces with the cool spring breeze. Stepping into the snow in August felt surreal. The hotel sat perched above the tree line, surrounded by a ring of towering peaks.

The terrain was wild—unmarked trails winding everywhere. After two days, we toyed with the idea of heliskiing—taking a helicopter to remote regions of the Andes to ski untouched powder—but the closer we got to booking, the riskier it felt.

Something in me had already begun to turn inward, trading adrenaline for stillness.

We walked up to the only convenience store within a 100-mile radius. In my broken Spanish, I asked for a pregnancy test. The woman behind the counter started jumping, her arms swinging high, hands clapping with a hip twist as she shuffled toward the shelves. She shouted something in rapid Spanish and I nodded like I understood, offering a quick smile. "Gracias," I said.

But it wouldn't have been a lie because when I walked into the restroom and peed on a stick, two pink lines grew. I went light-headed. I'd met Dave six months earlier. Could we really do this? I knew him, but how well can you know someone in six months? I stayed there for a moment, unsure for how long. I had thought about motherhood before, but never enough to stop me in my tracks. That's the thing about life—it can change direction in an instant.

The bright sun blinded me as I exited the lodge. I squinted as specks of light blurred into focus. Dave was sitting on a picnic table, his dark sunglasses covering his eyes, hiding whatever he felt. "Pregnant," I managed, holding up the flimsy plastic slip that revealed much more than a double line.

His smile grew. "No way." His voice filled with emotion. I was shaky. He leaned in and wrapped his arms around me, pulling me close. The steady beat of his heart calmed me.

I returned to the woman at the convenience store and asked for another test to be sure it wasn't lying. She jumped for joy again, just like the first time. She pointed at the test and said,

"Gemelos?" Her grin widened. Twins. I chuckled, as if tests worked that way. But something in her eyes made me pause. It was like she knew something I didn't.

Our exchanges went more on actions than words, but I could see the excitement in her eyes. And it was some reassurance that this journey wasn't to be feared.

We canceled the heliskiing trip and skied the mountain instead. The terrain hadn't changed, but mine had.

Risk didn't have to mean adrenaline. It could mean trust.

SEPTEMBER 2015

CHAUTAUQUA LAKE, NY

BLUE FOLDING INTO ORANGE

I went from skiing in the Andes to hurtling toward a wedding wrapped in fabric that clung tight.

Weeks ago, attending Dave's niece's wedding felt like an easy "yes." But the simplicity of that yes was unraveling with my fatigue, replaced by something more layered. A cocktail of anticipation rose—excitement tangled with uncertainty I couldn't yet name.

The hum of conversation wrapped around me, laughter rising, voices drifting between pleasantries. It was the same rhythm I had heard countless times before. The same questions. The same exchanges. But nothing felt the same.

Dave looked dapper in his suit and tie. I sipped my water, excitement heavy in my limbs. I listened, enjoying the easy rhythm of small talk, watching strangers drift between the weather and the passage of time—how quickly things change, don't they?

I glanced at the lake's setting sun, a kaleidoscope of blue and orange hues.

A voice beside me, casual, expectant. "So, what do you do, Tara?"

I blinked, looking up. The same question. Always.

"I am a nurse." I kept the talk small.

"Oh, what kind?"

And I thought of Maya, Tiny, Nancy, the ones who taught me about love and loss.

I had no answer. Not a real one.

The pause stretched between us.

How do I shrink something vast into something digestible?

I could feel everyone's eyes waiting for me to speak. I could feel the moment stretching, that invisible expectation of small talk and simple answers.

I adjusted the grip on my water glass.

"I'm an oncology nurse," I answered.

It's always the same.

The flicker of unease settled in, like it had before. Like it always did. The air shifted just slightly, that imperceptible moment when the weight of oncology drifts into a conversation that wasn't built for it.

The lake shimmered beside me. Blue folding into orange.

I LIKE THIS STORY

Selene jumped up when I walked in.

"How was Chile—ski the wild?" she asked, dropping whatever patient chart held her hostage. Few people matched Selene's appetite for adventure. Her latest trip was hiking Mt. Kilimanjaro. She'd burned through her PTO on earlier summits, once calling in sick from a satellite phone halfway up a mountain.

"Good morning to you, too, Selene." I laughed, sliding into my seat.

That made her pause. "Come on, for real. You're glowing, Duff!"

I smiled. "It was rugged. No trail markers, easy to get lost. And those crazy palma lifts kept launching me! I couldn't master them."

She smirked. "Third-world countries don't bother smoothing the edges. That's why they're worth the trip."

Her eyes sharpened, assessing me. "What was the best part?" Selene had a way of skirting the superficial.

I traced the rim of my Yeti. "Well...I'm pregnant."

The silence snapped into place.

Selene stared, then leaned back, arms crossing, recalibrating. "No way! Well, that's a hell of a plot twist."

I laughed, nervousness catching in my throat.

"This is exciting, Duff. I'm happy for you." There was a pause as her eyes narrowed, calculating. "You excited about this?"

I hesitated. "I'm excited, but it's moved fast. We met six months ago."

She watched me, considering. "Fast isn't necessarily bad. Fast means momentum. It's never about time. It's about trusting it."

I exhaled, then glanced upward. "Well, I trust it."

"That's how you know," she said with conviction.

I thought about that for far too long.

"Now you build it, like everything else worth holding onto."

I met her gaze, steady. "How'd you get so wise?"

She smiled. "It's oncology nursing; it changes us." She held the moment for a beat longer, then picked up the patient's chart and stood, already moving. "I like this story. Keep it going."

STEPPING STONES

Not every woman marked her life by the same milestones. Gail didn't, and something about that felt familiar, even in a borrowed room.

Gail never married, had no children, and didn't talk about those things as if they were tragedies. Gail was a 'float patient' to our floor because the GYN floor was overbooked for the day.

"Call me Gail," she said, squinting at my badge. Her eyes were deep blue and attentive, showing a presence that made me feel important.

"Oh, I am Tara," I apologized, flipping my badge around. "Sorry, my badge is always flipped, which is only fine when I am on the subway." I laughed at my joke. She studied me for a moment, as if taking in more than a badge.

"Well, what I really want to know is who you are, not the name your parents gave you."

I smiled, appreciating this shift from the small talk. "Oh, well, let's see then, I love nature, anything in it really—hiking, biking, skiing, I like writing and painting too. And my job, well I like this too." I chuckled again, nervously. I never liked conversations about me.

"Much better." She held a smile. Her voice was soft and soothing. "Husband? Kids?" There it was—the usuals.

"I am not married and have no kids." I wasn't sure what to call myself anymore.

"Oh, well, I pictured you with three little kids at home who adore you," she smiled. And I smiled back at her.

"Well, I am pregnant."

She smiled some more.

"You go, girl! Where are you hiding it?"

"Oh, it's here, all right," I pointed to a distended belly that looked like I was packing on the donuts.

She leaned into the conversation, her smile widening. "What are you having?" she asked, already invested in the unfolding story.

We tossed names back and forth, laughing at the ones that felt too bold or too bland. Gail liked old-fashioned names: Clara, June, Declan. I wasn't sure yet, but I liked how easily she joined the imagining.

Gail's demeanor shifted. "I never felt drawn toward children of my own."

Her tone turned heavy. I wondered: had I chosen motherhood, or simply let it happen? I've never been good at deliberation. Too much thinking and I lose the thread. Either way, I was excited for motherhood.

She continued, "My partner didn't either. I felt like it was what came next, and I wanted a better reason than that. I wanted a genuine, deep desire to be a mother beneath the stepping stones in life." She laughed. "I'm not one for stepping stones." Her eyes lightened, but something stayed unreadable.

I laughed, letting it land.

Gail's life was full—partner, friends, passions.

I found her firm stance on motherhood admirable. So many of us jump in headfirst without real thought as to why—myself included.

"I watched my friends and family members start families of their own. I saw the joy and fulfillment in their lives, and I was happy for them. I spoil my nieces and nephew and love being an aunt. But I never regretted my decision." Gail paused with curious, empathetic eyes, "I hope this isn't too close to home for you?"

"Not at all." I loved learning about others and our differences, especially those who colored outside the lines.

"How about you? Were you always drawn toward children of your own?" Her eyes were soft, unsure if she'd crossed a boundary.

I sighed, unsure myself. We often don't ask ourselves these questions. "Eh, I ebbed and flowed with it. I always thought it would just happen for me, actually." I paused, doubting my answer. "But the actual undertaking of motherhood? Not at all. I've always been someone who moves before I feel ready."

I gripped my fingers around my pen. Her pump's quiet churn filled the room, steady and unspoken. The kind of sound you stop hearing until you remember what it means.

"I don't even know what it means to be ready for motherhood."

We laughed.

"You have a refreshing presence."

I smirked.

"Hey, sometimes we need to just leap," Gail's chic bob swayed with her nod. "So, will you get married?" She loved a loaded question.

"We will, sometime before the baby is born."

With radiant eyes, Gail glanced at my belly and winked, "Oh, you've got time."

YOU'LL FLY

We met for lunch near the hospital, a tiny café tucked between scaffolding and more scaffolding. Meg was already there when I arrived, her coat draped over the back of her chair, a mug of tea warming her hands.

"I'm fasting," she said, smiling. "But I'll watch you eat."

I laughed, lowering myself into the chair with the kind of effort that made strangers offer help.

"Thankfully, fasting isn't allowed when you're pregnant." I was very pregnant, hips aching, belly taut, breath shallow. I ordered soup and bread, something warm and simple. Meg sipped her tea.

We hadn't seen each other in months, but it didn't matter. With Meg, the conversation always picked up mid-sentence, like we'd just paused to laugh.

"How are you?" she asked, eyes steady.

I shrugged. "Tired. Excited. You?"

"Just starving. No room for anything else."

She salivated, watching me butter a piece of bread.

"What's it like? Being this close to becoming someone's mother?"

I paused, the question landing somewhere deep. I looked down at my meal, then back at Meg.

"Great question. No one's asked me that yet—they've only spilled out random advice." We laughed. And Meg waited—for a real answer.

"I guess it's kinda like standing on a cliff," I said. "Everyone tells you the views are beautiful, but you're still afraid of the fall."

Meg didn't flinch. She just nodded, like she'd stood on her own cliff once or twice. A smile rose to her lips as her hands wrapped around the mug like it was something sacred. "You'll fly."

I wanted to believe her. I wanted to believe I could hold space for patients and a baby, for grief and joy, for the woman I was and the one I was becoming. But I didn't say that. I just took another bite of bread and let her presence anchor me, the way only an old friend can when life is tilting toward something new.

TUESDAY AT 12:15

On our first of many chairlift rides together, Dave asked, "Would you consider pursuing a guy my age?"

"I would. I enjoy your company. For me, that's half the battle."

"What's the other half?"

"It's a feeling."

Dave nodded, playing it cool.

As an oncology nurse for a few years, I knew death was the only guarantee in life. I also knew the odds of a longer life partner would be better if I married someone closer to my age. But in my line of work, I saw the spread.

I didn't use this logic before I married Dave, though; I went on feeling. I knew better than to fight love. Love always wins.

On the day we got married, my belly arrived before I did. We did the courthouse thing. I called on a Tuesday. "Let's see," I heard the woman tapping the computer keys on the other side of the line. "We do weddings on Tuesdays. I have a wedding at 12:10 p.m. next Tuesday, February 2nd; how about 12:15?" It was Groundhog Day, and conveniently, Dave would be in town. "Perfect," I said, ending the call and feeling nothing I could name. It felt like stepping into a life I hadn't fully caught up to yet.

Dave felt strongly about being married before the baby arrived, and I liked the idea too. Per my parents' love and wishes, we would have a wedding ceremony, but I tabled it till after the baby's arrival.

The magistrate called us forward. She was stern and plump; it didn't look like she smiled much.

"IDs, please," she demanded.

I immediately realized mine was home in my nursing backpack.

"Uhhh, I forgot mine," I said. "We—"

"I will vouch for her—she is my daughter," my mom cut me off, handing over her license, and I felt a wave of gratitude wash over me. Grateful, as always, for my mother.

The magistrate must've felt it, because something in her expression loosened.

"Well, if you say you are who you are, let's take your vows." And so we did. She declared us husband and wife within two minutes.

WHEN A FLOOR WAS HOME

As I placed my backpack in my cubby, Kylie approached me without pause.

"Good morning, Tara. Did you get married?"

I smiled at her uncanny timing. Kylie had a way of knowing before I said a word.

The team of thoracic nurses stood behind her, pretending to be busy, ears tuned in.

"Yesterday," I said with an uncomfortable smile. I never liked attention. Heads turned, voices rose, and suddenly the nurses were all talking at once—asking for pictures, wanting the Groundhog Day story. I pulled up our one picture. "Oh, Tara, that is so special," Laura said, pointing to my belly.

"I love the blue dress," added Raya, as Selene and Tony whispered behind the crowd.

The phone rang, and Tony answered. "It's GYN; a patient wants you to stop by."

"Me?"

"They said Tara," Tony repeated. I thought about Elsa or Gail and appreciated the escape from the spotlight.

I headed downstairs.

The nurses pointed me toward the room ahead. I slid the curtain open, revealing Gail.

"Whoa, you got big!" Gail's chic bob bounced with her heavy nod, unaware of her insensitivity. I laughed; people said all kinds of things about a pregnant belly.

"I got married." I nodded, knowing Gail would be eager for my latest life update.

Gail's smile grew as she pulled my hand in closer. "Where's the ring?"

I sat beside Gail, my hips aching beneath me. Pregnancy had turned even small movements into effort.

"I didn't wear it—I was afraid I'd lose it with all the gloves I peeled off each day."

"It's that big?" Gail smirked.

It was beautiful, but I never wanted a ring. I'd take skis or a vacation instead.

"No." I grew flushed, embarrassed by the superficiality. But it mattered to Dave.

"Hey—I brought you a little something," Gail said, pulling up a gift bag from beneath her chemo chair. I pulled off the tissue paper. On top was a musical stuffed lamb and the children's book, *City Dog, Country Frog.*

"Oh, Gail, this is so sweet of you," I said, moved by her thoughtfulness.

"Here, turn this," she said. The lamb started playing the tune of *Somewhere Over the Rainbow.* Its soft, soothing rhythm tugged at something early in me, from before I had words for the world. "And this is one of my favorite books," Gail paused. "I read it to my nephews." Something in her pause made the room feel briefly suspended.

"Thank you so much, Gail; what is it about?" I asked.

"A city dog and a country frog," she said with a small smirk that tugged on my heart. Something in her tone made me aware of time again. I had a few weeks left at MSK but wasn't ready to part with any of it. I thanked Gail for the thoughtful gifts and hugged her goodbye. It's a particular kind of goodbye, hugging someone you've known only in this place, in this season. "I want to see baby pictures! Here is my email," Gail said as we stepped apart.

When I reentered Thoracic 9, the back counter at the nurses' station was lined with pink and blue frosted cupcakes—compliments of the team I would soon be leaving.

"We are going to drive to Pittsburgh when you're in labor," Selene said, straight-faced.

There was a rhythm to Thoracic 9—an ease, a way of moving together that felt rare. Tony filmed a snippet from a sneaky angle on his phone, but the video only caught a fraction of the beauty. The rest shimmered just beyond language.

Leaving that floor felt like stepping out of a world I wasn't ready to lose. But chapters close whether we're ready or not, and mine was already unfolding.

I lingered in the pace of the place. I didn't know how to say goodbye. So, I kept clocking in, kept showing up, until my story moved on.

PART IV

2016—PITTSBURGH, PA

UPMC HILLMAN CANCER CENTER

SHE FELT SO HEAVY

Labor felt like something breaking open from the inside. Light burned through my eyelids. My head throbbed. Each contraction pulled me deeper into the churning undertow. I desperately wanted to escape the pain. Each contraction was searing, primal—the universe focused entirely on me.

"A hundred percent effaced," the doctor shouted at 9 a.m. Labor had started at 5. My legs spread, gown flowing open, revealing everything I'd learned to cover. Dave stood beside me, steady but helpless.

"I want an epidural!" I snapped at the kind nurse handing me an exercise ball.

Bent over the bed, I kicked the birthing ball and felt a brief, useless flicker of relief. The anesthesiologist told me I needed to stay very still while he slid the long needle into my spine. "We don't want to cause damage," he said, almost bored. I wanted to punch him, but instead, I sat frozen, trembling inside. The needle terrified me—but not as much as another hour with that birthing ball.

The relief was instantaneous, rushing through my spine and dispersing like warm water over ice. I sighed loudly and rested, grateful for the pause. For a moment, the room felt hushed, as if everyone was waiting with me.

But labor doesn't wait.

Soon, voices rose again, urgent and insistent, pulling me back into the storm.

"No, no—push on the exhale," she said, her voice firm but full of care. Our first encounter was in the blur and noise of labor. Fierce and composed—exactly what I needed. Yet her instructions were a fragmented echo in my mind. On my inhale, I pushed.

Beside me, Dave rubbed my arm, his chuckle breaking through the tension. "You're pushing at the wrong time." Heat flushed my face, and my blood pressure surged—my now-husband offering birthing advice. I couldn't muster more than an "Umph." A flash of heat moved through me, just enough to push past the final threshold.

The crying pierced the air as relief surged through me, bypassing every ache and landing in my chest. Our baby had arrived.

Euphoria settled in as the tumult ebbed. I was sweating, shivering, and smiling. Ruined and remade, all at once. Something in me had already changed, even before I understood what it meant.

I wanted to hold my newborn immediately, but the doctor needed to stitch up some of my vaginal tears, and the thought distracted me. It felt like I was underwater, my crying baby muffled and distant. My ears rang, my vision tunneled. I asked for my baby. For water. For warmth.

The room spun as I floated on a cloud of relief and exhaustion. Everything blurred—scrubs, hats, movement. The room seemed to expand and tilt.

Maybe that's how motherhood begins—not with clarity, but with blur. And for the first time, I understood what it felt like to be the one in the bed, not the one standing beside it.

"It's a girl!" someone yelled.

"A girl?" I mustered.

"You seem surprised," the nurse said, all smiles.

I was.

I waited for them to bring my baby to me. It was in the birth plan, the same one I'd handed my doctor weeks ago. She took it with a smile, though we joked later that birth plans were more ceremonial than practical.

They placed my new daughter in a little pink hat and brought her to me. I held her outside my body for the first time. Our skin touched—her warm little body against my chest, my arms wrapped around her. Her legs pressed against my belly, as if trying to restore it to what it was.

She felt so heavy, this little thing, a life in my arms to love and protect. Her big blue eyes opened for the first time, looking up at me. A rush moved through me, the kind that changes you in an instant—like something inside me sparked and took shape.

LIFE IS BUT A DREAM

Everything felt shifted, as if the sun rose differently now. And in Pittsburgh, people rearranged their days to catch its rare light after a long winter. But sunrise no longer marked beginnings for me. My days were a run-on sentence—nights melting into days, days dissolving into nights. I turned the lamb's key and pulled Addison (who we mostly called Addy) to my breast, already emptied out in that new-mother way. Her nursing slowed to the soft tune of *Row, Row, Row Your Boat*. The melody floated, woozy by nature, and so was I. Childhood seeped in without words, only rhythm. It was bone-deep exhaustion, yet a new, unfamiliar contentment settled in—one that felt deeply mine. Like waking from a dream so peaceful you want to close your eyes and return. Life is but a dream.

HILLMAN

UPMC didn't shape me the way other places did; it simply carried me through a season when I was becoming someone else. I had a newborn, a new marriage, a new city. My life outside the hospital was full in a way it had never been, and the nursing job—for the first time—was just a job. At MSK, I felt like part of something. At UPMC, I felt like a part. I wasn't mistreated, just counted. I was "casual," or per diem, so I swiped in and out. Full-time nurses were salaried, their extra hours absorbed into the culture without acknowledgment. Stay late. Be flexible.

It was a solid-tumor floor—lung, breast, pancreatic, GI, head and neck—and the difference wasn't the pace, but the feel of the place. The atmosphere was sterile, jaundiced light replacing sun. Even the curtains snagged my computer. Nothing moving easily. The nurses were busy. Chemotherapy required a second nurse to cosign, which happened from the desk—streamlined, but different from what I was used to, where we cross-checked with the patient too.

Addison—Addy—loved her breastmilk and hated sleeping

alone, part temperament, part me still learning how to mother. I was tired, and pumping was a priority.

I asked my nurse manager where I could pump. "Pump?" She blinked, as if I'd asked about a hospital petting zoo. Without looking up, she said, "I think there's a station. Across the bridge." She shuffled a stack of papers. With a rare 20-minute lunch, pumping was a puzzle missing pieces.

A couple of weeks in, a manager approached me. "You'll need to clock out when you pump."

"Can't I use my lunch?" I asked.

She fidgeted with her pen, like it might answer for her. "You can pump. We don't pay for that time."

It was such a small sentence, but it told me everything. I walked away.

It made me question if I belonged. I hadn't expected anything to change. I'd always nudged for clarity in small ways, trying to hold the line where I could. I knew what care felt like when there was room for it.

That afternoon, another manager stopped by.

"You can pump without clocking out." I nodded, grateful for the gesture. But the bruise had already formed. The moment had already settled into me, an underscore of this new and different kind of place. It wasn't MSK, and I knew better than to search for pearls in sand. What felt the same, though, were the patients.

A DIFFERENT KIND OF ROAD

Jack wore a dangling earring, a toothpick between his teeth, tattoos peeking through his cutoff tee. Mischievous eyes hinted at the rest.

"I just got back from Colorado—rode my bike there," he said, minutes into our meeting.

"Wow, that must have been challenging." The small talk eased nerves, lightening the intensity of cancer for a moment.

"Well, I was with some buddies," he said, rolling the toothpick between his teeth.

"How long did that take you?"

"We did it in a week—we do it every year." I pictured him pedaling through golden aspens until his wife, Carol, caught my look.

"On a motorcycle."

"Ohhh," I laughed, realizing my confusion. "I thought you meant pedal bike."

Jack looked at me dubiously, half a smirk forming at the edges of his mouth.

It was his first treatment—stage IV non-small cell lung

cancer. His plan was indefinite, treatment continuing as long as the drugs slowed growth—what we call "responding."

"I started motorcycling as a way to soul search," he said, eyes softening for just a beat. Carol smiled, her gaze knowing. The conversation shifted the way it often did in these rooms away from their pain and toward my life instead. She turned to me, warm and expectant. "Do you have a family?"

I hesitated. I had people I called my family now, but the question still felt too neat.

"I have a four-month-old daughter," I finally said, the warmth of Addison threading through me.

"Oh, how sweet." Carol pressed on. "A husband?"

"Yes, I'm married. Actually, we're celebrating next weekend."

"A wedding?"

"We got married in February, just a courthouse thing. My parents wanted a proper wedding after the baby arrived, and honestly, I liked the idea too."

Carol's face lit up. Jack remained impassive, his gaze drifting.

"Oh, lovely! Will the baby be in it?" The questions tumbled out.

I did my best to field them but felt the contrast of weddings and new beginnings in a room built for managing endings.

Jack looked down, then up again. The pause said more than words could.

Some moments remain heavy, no matter how others try to lift them.

HERE'S TO THE MOMENTS

Ed arrived late to my wedding. He seemed to materialize with the breeze alongside Shannon, mid-speech. Ed—Maureen's husband, the one who had barreled through my MSK years—lingered just long enough to unsettle before breaking in.

"Done yet?" Ed interrupted.

Shannon stiffened, her speech still in hand. "I'm sorry—*who* are you?"

"Here, give me that mic," Ed said, reaching for it.

Dave leaned in. "Who the hell is this guy?"

My pulse quickened; I whispered, "My patient's husband, Ed. I wasn't sure he'd come." I tried to stay calm, knowing Maureen would've reeled him in. She had passed away just months prior. Her prognosis was always bleak, but that didn't make my heart any less heavy.

Ed took the mic, commanding the room. He paused, and the noise fell away.

"This night started with something small," Ed began. "Tonight's a big moment—weddings, vacations, births. But the small ones? The ones when we actually listen—not just to people we know, but to strangers whose words end up reshaping us."

The crowd shifted, a ripple of confusion moving through the room. No one quite knew what I knew. To them, he was a wedding crasher or a drunk uncle. To me, he was Maureen's husband—the man whose grief had once spilled into my workdays at MSK.

"I told Tara about Big Sky, Montana," he continued, pulling a trail map from his back pocket. I let out a chuckle—his signature move always landed somewhere between charm and prophecy.

"Sometimes it's just small talk. Other times, one conversation changes everything."

He took a breath, steadying himself.

"Here's to the moments we don't see coming—the ones that carry us exactly where we're meant to go."

Applause rose, glasses clinked. "Hear, hear."

Ed parted through the cluster of guests, eyes locked on Dave.

Dave was all smiles, extending his hand. "Dave," he said warmly. "Nice to finally meet you."

Ed, cold and stoic, gripped Dave's hand tight.

"Don't fuck this up." Ed's grip didn't loosen. His eyes stayed on Dave, unreadable.

I stepped in, breaking the tension with a stiff embrace. Just awkward enough to feel familiar.

"His last name is Wed—*more*?"

"It is," I smirked.

"Better not be any *more* wed—dings after this one." Ed shifted his gaze from Dave to me. My face softened, realizing we were missing someone. "Ed, I'm so sorry about Maureen. I wish she could have been here." I needed to say her name. She was the reason our worlds had collided at all.

"Thank you. Maureen would have loved to be here," Ed said, his voice catching, a small crack he couldn't hide. It was the first time he let something raw slip through. "Where are you skiing this winter?" he redirected, and Dave felt the comfort of ski talk soften the space between them.

Ed wanted the night to be about life. And when I thought about it, all my encounters with Ed and Maureen had been about living—skiing the finest mountains, making work meaningful, finding someone to love.

Through the hum of conversation and clinking glasses, the opening chords of a Dierks Bentley song rose above the room, and I felt its meaning settle deep in my bones the way certain songs do when life is shifting.

"And don't fucking lose this." Ed gripped Dave's hand, pressing an envelope into it.

Dave forced a smile, a nervous chuckle escaping. I let the song carry me, sensing the quiet alignment in that strange collision of worlds.

Ed danced the night away, flirting shamelessly with all the women and telling his part in our story to anyone who would listen. Eventually, he disappeared into the late night without much of a goodbye. We tried to keep in touch, but he distanced himself immediately. Without Maureen, it was as if his role in my life had already been fulfilled. Maybe that was always how it was meant to be—a fleeting but meaningful presence, stepping in just long enough to change everything.

Some moments feel small when they happen, but eventually, we see them for what they are: the beginning of everything and the subtle ending of what came before.

THEY BOTH LOOKED SO VIBRANT

The sky hung heavy, mirroring my mood. One day, she will sleep through the night, I told myself as I unloaded Addison, Rocky, and the gear from the Jeep. The morning was crisp, though sweat was already rising through my skin.

It was my favorite spot up the hill from our townhouse—Dark Hollow. The oak trees created a canopy, their branches interwoven like protective arms. Fallen leaves carpeted the path, crunching underfoot. The fall foliage was at its peak. I carried Addy in the baby carrier on my chest, facing outward. The fiery red and orange branches overhead caught her awe. When I was open to it—when I let her wonder slow me—she brought me there too. We stood still, taking in the colors. I wondered if the leaves still holding on knew what was coming, if they understood they'd soon join the ones beneath my feet. They looked so vibrant.

I walked down to the ravine. It wove between two hillsides, splitting them with rocky streams and arching bridges. I was on one of the bridges with no rails when my phone rang. Maya scrolled across my screen. I was nervous but eager to hear from her. Last I heard, she was doing outpatient chemotherapy—they found 20% blast cells in her bone marrow. In other words, relapse.

"Maya!" I answered.

Something in the silence told me it wasn't her.

"Hi Tara, it's Carly." My eyes welled; my chin quivered.

"She's gone, Tara. Maya passed." Carly's words trailed off with the November breeze. The truth hit in pieces, slow and sharp."Thank you for being the light to us during this dark time," Carly said, her voice catching.

Tears streamed down my face, landing on Addy's pink hat below. She looked upward, babbling as my breath caught.

I cried for a friend I barely knew, but somehow knew deeply.

"I am so sorry, Carly," I said, my voice shaky.

"Maya loved you like a friend," Carly said.

"I did, too. I loved her too. I wish I could have explored with her outside the hospital," I managed, barely getting the words out.

"In another life," Carly added as I looked down at Addy, her pink hat bright against the gray morning. I pressed on with the hike, the urge to climb taking over, as if distance could lessen the ache. I veered off the path onto the steep hillside. Grief climbed with me, impossible to shake. I should've reach out sooner, but I didn't. I guess I thought we had more time.

At the peak, my breath finally caught. I pulled Addy from the carrier, her heavy little body settling into my arms. I kissed her chubby cheek. "I love you—I will love you more than you ever know," I mustered, grief and gratitude tangled in my chest.

The sky looked less gray. Leaves circled around with the invisible wind currents. I picked up a bright orange leaf and placed the stem in Addy's hand. She lit up with delight, waving it toward her open-mouthed smile.

They both looked so vibrant.

WEIGHTED VEST

At 82, she sat upright and spoke in an uplifting voice. "Aging isn't easy, but it's not like we have a choice," she chuckled.

A rare lull in my schedule gave me room to linger, and something about Miss June made me want to.

"It's always in how we look at things, Miss Tara," she said, biting into her apple.

"It is all about perspective, isn't it?" A perspective I reached for more often than I ever caught.

"Oh, yes." She smiled softly, as if remembering something. "Do you have children, Miss Tara?"

"I have a daughter," I said. "She'll be one in May. When I'm not here, she's on my hip."

"Wonderful. Enjoy that little smoosh. You never get enough time with your children." Her expression warmed. "That baby will grow on you and have her own hopes and dreams. It will be challenging in new ways."

I tried to imagine Addy with dreams of her own, but all I could picture was her reaching for me. Maybe that was the beginning of it.

"When my Johnny was little—I used to think, Lord, how am

I going to survive this stage? He was wild. Curious. Always running ahead of me."

She laughed. "But now? I'd give anything to chase after him again. Time moves fast, Miss Tara. Faster than you think. Enjoy that hip hugger."

I leaned in, unsure at first what she meant. Most of my days were spent with Addy, and I craved growth—the kind where sleep returned and my arms weren't always full. Then again, maybe holding her was the growth.

"Now he gifts me weighted vests," she said, laughing. "As if I'm not slow enough already."

"I am slower, and my joints ache, but my body still needs to move. Oh, he's probably right."

"The beach has changed for me over the years," she said. "It used to be swimming with my siblings, then chasing my children, and now it's just walking the shoreline." She lifted a finger, smirking. "With my weighted vest now."

"Have you ever walked on a beach with snow?"

I smiled. "No, I imagine that'd be beautiful."

"Oh, beautiful indeed." Her eyes brightened. "It fills me with wonder. I always make a snow angel. You can't make a snow angel without smiling."

I tried to remember the last time I'd made a snow angel. I couldn't. I couldn't remember the last time I'd done something just for the wonder of it. And yet, somehow, Addison kept nudging me back toward wonder.

"It took me a while," she said, "but one day, I finally felt at home in my own skin."

I didn't know what to say, so I said nothing.

"When you look in the mirror," she added, "those faint lines on your face—let them be a celebration."

Heat tightened my chest. I thought about the Botox party invite I'd declined. "Were you always able to do that?"

She laughed, loud and whole. "Oh, Lord, no. Only when I

started yearning for my youth. But now I honor those feelings. I let them pass. I was young once. I lived that life. It's my turn to be this age."

"I like that," I said, and meant it.

She mentioned fatigue once or twice, but she didn't dwell on it. The treatment was part of her life now, not the center of it.

Outside the door, the call bells started up again. I stepped away knowing that when I returned, the window for this kind of honesty might close.

As we parted, she looked at me, her eyes bright with something both young and ancient.

"Remember, Miss Tara," she said, "embrace the journey, every day of it."

I nodded, unsure if I could but wanting to try.

BECAUSE THEY NO LONGER CAN

She was about my age.

A snowboarder.

A mother.

Her name was Taylor.

"I'm not strong enough anymore," she said when I asked about snowboarding.

Taylor was late in her cancer journey by the time we met. Another drug had failed her. She spoke with a finality, like someone who had folded away part of herself, tucked it into a drawer with clothes that would never fit again.

We were nearly the same age. Both mothers. Both once stood atop a mountain, heart pounding, board strapped to our feet, staring down a long stretch of winter. I don't remember how we got on the subject. It wasn't ski season yet, but I was already counting snow before it fell.

Embarrassment flushed through me. Taylor could barely stand, and here I was expecting snow like it was promised.

Grief ached in my chest for something neither of us could fix. Yet I hung a bag of chemotherapy, as if treating the end could rewrite the beginning.

Taylor had children. Their ages didn't stick in my memory the way the rest of her story did. A boyfriend who sometimes sat with her. She still had so much tethering her to this world. But cancer doesn't tally that up before it takes.

Taylor died not long after that conversation. But her words stayed with me. Not with pity, but with reverence. Because maybe that's the only way to keep carrying someone after they go—by feeling everything a little deeper, because they no longer can.

WE SETTLE INTO IT

Evening settled like a soft exhale, the kind that seeps into your bones. Pittsburgh and motherhood still had their unknowns, but evenings felt like mine. Addy breathed steadily through the monitor. Rocky glanced up from the couch, then dropped his head again with a thud. Dave was traveling for work. I stood in the kitchen, hands wrapped around a glass of water, everything finally still.

Marriage. A baby. A new city. All of it came in such a rush, like being swept into a current I didn't know I'd stepped into. I had spent the last year catching my breath. But somewhere in the blur, rhythm arrived. Diapers and white noise. The click of infusion pumps. Dave's laugh from the other room—movement without resistance.

And yet, some silences are different.

At MSK, I never had to go looking for noise. Blunt honesty from down the hall. Deadpan storytelling. Mischief. Maternal check-ins. We talked about everything and nothing in the same breath. I missed it all. The way it cracked me open and stitched me back together in the same shift. That chatter had been a kind of oxygen.

At UPMC, the culture was more careful. Still competent, but fewer moments slipped past my guard mid-shift. And yet, the patients still found me. Still offered those profound flashes of humanity. I still bore witness.

I sipped my water and curled up beside Rocky, thinking of Miss June's voice from just the day before. Her words stuck with me: "We don't escape change. We settle into it."

I looked down the hallway toward Addy's room. Then at Rocky, his eyes barely opening as I patted him. Another new home for the two of us. But it no longer felt hollow. Somewhere in time, somehow, it became home.

Change once felt jarring. Now it felt like rhythm.

THE CANCELED TRIP

His name was Rich. Sixty-seven, sharp-witted, the kind of dry humor that made you lean in. He was being treated for colorectal cancer. But he wore his prognosis like a loose jacket —shrugged on, never zipped.

It was late spring when we met. We'd just started treatment, and he was sitting upright in his chair, scrolling through photos on his phone.

"We were going to Alaska," he said, eyes still on the screen. "Cruise up the Inside Passage. I wanted to see icebergs before I became one."

He chuckled, but it scraped the air. "My wife and I talked about it for years. Every anniversary, we'd say—'Next, when we've got more time.' Then the kids' weddings. Then retirement. Then this."

He gestured toward the IV pole. "Funny how easily the years drift past while we're busy planning for them."

I asked if they'd booked anything.

He nodded. "Reservations, itinerary, the works. Canceled it all when I started chemo. Figured we'd wait until I felt stronger." A pause. "We'll see if that's coming."

His voice didn't shake, but something in me did.

When I left the room, I couldn't stop thinking about it. The unused tickets. The hikes he'd never take. The parts of Alaska he'd already let go of.

JULY 4TH, TAHOE

We skied Tahoe on the Fourth of July.

It was hot enough in town to wear tank tops, but we chased the melting snow. Dave and I rode the lift past patches of green, the mountain clinging to its last veins of summer slush.

Addison stayed with my parents, who didn't hesitate, because to them, love is a reflex.

That trip wouldn't have happened years earlier. But working in cancer care changes your relationship to hesitation. You stop waiting for the perfect conditions. You go. Because the moment is now. And you've seen too many people lose their Someday.

We wore sunglasses instead of goggles. Skied in T-shirts. The snow was mushy and melting fast, but it held just long enough. We got sunburned. It was beautiful, ridiculous summer snow.

But it wasn't about the skiing.

It was about doing something just because we were alive.

WHERE THE HAWK CIRCLES

The foliage lined the Allegheny River far below us, meandering through the valley. A sea of summer green with splashes of crimson. Dave and I were on a late summer hike a few days after we found out I was pregnant. It was my 36th birthday.

The sun pierced my vision like a thousand tiny needles. I blinked, and the dream from the night before surfaced.

"I had a crazy dream last night," I blurted, wanting to reveal it before it slipped back into the shadows of my mind.

"A coworker...Colleen," I said, drawing the dream from my subconscious. "She handed me two blue gifts. I asked, 'Oh, I'm having a boy?' She said, 'You don't know? You're having two.'"

Dave smiled faintly. "Oh boy."

We kept climbing.

We summited the grueling steep, my breath coming fast. A weathered bench awaited us. The air felt thick. The river stretched wide, its surface rippling like molten silver. Farther upstream, a bridge spanned high above the water, a slender thread connecting two worlds.

"Beautiful view," Dave said.

A hawk circled, held up by currents I couldn't see. Maybe he'd grown numb to his bird's-eye view.

"It sure is."

And that was that. No more questions.

It was just a dream, after all.

ABOVE THE BODY

Life kept moving, my body changing. My mind felt fogged, unsteady. And in the midst of it all, I met Amir.

Nausea came in waves, each one dragging me under like a riptide. I let a cracker dissolve on my tongue, the brief relief gone as the next surge rose. It was hard to feel sick and put others first.

To fight the urge to fold into the nearest bed.

To meet the needs of others who felt ill too.

This is just temporary, I told myself as I walked into Amir's room.

His eyes were closed. His lashes fluttered. Jealousy pricked at me. I wished I could lie down. But the list awaited: introduce myself, start an IV, and attend to three other patients.

"Good morning, Amir," I said gently.

He opened his eyes, unstartled.

"Good morning," he replied—alert, pleasant.

"I'm Tara. I apologize for waking you—"

"Am-ir," he interrupted, voice steady. "I was not asleep. I was not in my body."

I stopped.

For the first time all morning, I slowed.

Unsure how to respond, I asked quietly, "Where were you?"

Amir chuckled. "Above my body, watching everything from the outside looking in. Meditation," he added.

The rush of the morning dissipated.

I liked meditation but never carved the space in my day. And there was Amir, practicing what I had never managed to begin.

"Well, how do I go there?" I asked. "I'd love to learn."

"What would you like to know?"

"How to escape discomfort?" I chuckled.

Amir held a smile. "It takes a lot of practice, Tara. You need to get into the body to get out of the mind."

"But what if it isn't in my head?"

He laughed softly. "I can't escape discomfort. I sit beside it."

His words circled back:

To get out of the mind, you had to stay in the body.

Even when it hurt.

I exhaled, nauseous.

"If only we all had that strength."

"We do. But you need not be too busy to learn." He winked.

"Give me one quick lesson," I joked.

Amir chuckled. "Start by breathing in through the left lung and nostril, out on the right."

I inhaled on my left side, handing Amir his medication.

"Is that even possible?" I exhaled. Both lungs released.

Amir winked, eyes closing.

I kept breathing, nausea retreating with each slow inhale.

"You're getting it," Amir whispered, eyes still closed.

Amir had lung cancer. He was responding incredibly well to treatment.

I stood there, practicing unilateral breathing long enough to glimpse the quiet he lived in.

Amir stayed with his breath.

I returned to my list, envying him more than I cared to admit.

A DOUBLE MIRACLE

We went to the 12-week nuchal translucency test, recommended because of my advanced maternal age. The room was dim and clinical. Dave, Addison, and I paused in the doorway, letting our pupils adjust. It smelled like every hospital morning I'd ever known; machines hummed in the silence.

The ultrasound tech guided us in, her expression tight. "Please lie here," she said, applying icy gel to my bulging abdomen, sending a shiver through me.

She circled the cold knob. Her brows lifted. A flicker of something unfamiliar—excitement?

"Hmm . . ." she said, her tone catching me off guard. "How would you feel about two babies?"

I lay there awestruck. The words came soft but sank like stones in still water.

"Wait—what?"

She smiled at me for the first time all morning. "You are growing two babies. I see two babies."

"Wow," I managed, goosebumps rising throughout my limbs as I replayed my dream.

Addy started crying—a cry too loud for the space. At one, she only wanted to climb into my lap. "Momma."

Dave's face lost its coloring. "Your dream . . ." he managed.

"There is something concerning here. I'd like you to meet with a doctor."

She ran off to find the doctor. Silence stretched—thick, suffocating, heavy with questions no one could answer.

Everything happened at once and not at all. The babies were still growing inside me, exactly as before. And yet we were caught in a whirlwind of worry, grasping for answers faster than anyone could give them. But there were none to give.

Appointments followed—genetic counselors, high-risk OBGYNs, cardiologists.

I'd been in rooms like these before—but never with my own child's heart on the screen.

Dr. T., a high-risk OBGYN known for handling complex cases, saw us first thing the next morning. She stood like a pillar beneath her white coat, poised and blunt.

"I don't sugarcoat things."

I nodded, palms sweating, heart racing. It felt like I was hit by a wave, searching for the sand.

"These numbers scare me. When I see this, I am concerned." She spoke her mind. "This heart is so tiny and intricate. It's a miracle when things go right."

Her eyes held mine, unwavering. Her words morphed into a distant, muffled echo, as if I were underwater and she was speaking from the shore.

Between her inaudible concerns, I went somewhere else. Somewhere quiet. Inward.

In the silence of that place, the possibility of a double miracle surfaced.

I understood my patients' silence differently after that.

THE SPACE BETWEEN

The babies shared a placenta. If one was high-risk, they both were. One could not survive without the other. Mono-di twins: one placenta, two sacs. Likely identical, but not definitive.

The doctors recommended an amniocentesis. I asked if there were other options. I pictured the needle, the risk unfolding in slow motion like a film reel I couldn't stop. I couldn't do it.

My instinct answered before I could. Faith was becoming something tangible—something I could hold onto. I heeded the science, but I held on to instinct.

At 36, I fell into the category of advanced maternal age, which meant I qualified for a genetic blood test. It wasn't risky —just a peripheral draw that would analyze the babies' DNA and screen for common genetic abnormalities, especially the one they suspected.

As they drew the sample from my arm, I said a prayer to God and all the angels I've collected along the way.

I may never know where faith ends and science begins. But in that space between, I held on to hope and instinct.

THE NEW TEACH

In oncology, we call first-time patients a "New Teach."

By happenstance, Siena became my patient.

It felt larger than coincidence.

There was something about her. A quiet fierceness. She walked like she didn't need anyone's approval, which somehow made me want hers.

Her husband trailed behind her, arms full of bags. But Siena was the one who took up space.

"I don't want to know anything about the drugs or the side effects," she said coolly as she unpacked a book I couldn't quite catch the title of. Her voice was firm. Unapologetic.

Siena motioned toward the door. "You can teach my husband somewhere else." Siena had been diagnosed with a cancer she met with a quiet fierceness. She'd found a small bump along her neckline. Nothing in her posture betrayed it. She didn't spiral into a hundred questions. She chose not to drown in the "what ifs." Not knowing was her armor.

Siena and I barely spoke during her infusion. I respected her boundaries. She read while her chemo dripped, one leg crossed elegantly over the other, eyes flicking up only when necessary.

I leaned in to check her IV. The smell of antiseptic and adhesive tape turned my stomach again, sharper than usual.

"You okay?" Siena asked, glancing up from her journal.

"Yeah," I lied with a forced smile.

She raised a brow. "What are you having?" she asked.

I exhaled, feeling relieved to share with someone. “Twins.”

She smiled. "I carried twins."

I looked up.

"Twice."

BLACK, WHITE, BLUE

Addy and I skipped. Leaves swirled in the wind. My phone rang. It was the genetic counselor. Her name never stuck. I pictured her flipping through my results, her ruler-thick Book of Worries at her side.

"Mrs. Wedmore"—a name that never felt like mine. My heart was racing, palms slick, toddler in hand, and I tried to wear calm like something borrowed.

"The test results came back," she said, then paused.

Paused like it was helpful. Like she was telling me about her grocery list.

"And…no detectable genetic abnormalities!"

Relief washed over me. She kept talking, "This doesn't mean they don't have a genetic abnormality; we just test for the most common . . ." but my mind drifted elsewhere. A weight I hadn't even noticed had lifted. "We also know the babies' sex now, which will be attached in an email . . ." I sighed, eager for the conversation to end.

Addy pulled at my arm, and I swung her onto my hip. I skipped to the playground, her little voice sounding more vibrant, the gray sky seeming brighter. Even the wind felt gentler, as if it had been holding its breath with me. I filled my lungs with the cool autumn air and basked in the faint glow of sunlight breaking through.

I saw her email the next day at work. "Sensitive information," the email subject line read. The anticipation coiled in my chest, a mix of curiosity and trepidation. No pink-and-blue cake, no golf ball bursting with color, no waiting crowd. Just stark reality delivered in black and white. Exactly the way I wanted it. I clicked.

Male. Male.

Boys.

The words landed heavy, electric. A heat rose behind my sternum, the kind that feels like a fuse catching. And my nose tingled—the sensation you get right before tears that never fully come.

I leaned back in my creaky chair, staring through the window into the gray sky. The world carried on, oblivious to the shift inside me.

Two boys. I held the words in my chest like a spark. Not a reveal, not a spectacle—just a new shape to my future. A new kind of love already forming.

Outside, the wind stirred the trees. Inside, I sat still.

BETWEEN HOPE AND REALITY

She approached, her eyes speaking before her lips moved. "Someone needs to talk to my mom; she's living out of touch with reality."

I exhaled. "I can help you with that."

The daughter smiled, tears in her eyes. "She keeps telling my brother Dad's not in pain, that he can walk. But it took three people to get him out of the car and into the wheelchair. He has suffered enough."

I nodded. No convincing was needed.

Her mother hovered close, holding tight to a hope her daughter had already let go of.

I was the treating nurse for her father, Frank. At 78, he lay curled in the treatment chair, his discomfort palpable. Two other nurses and I repositioned him twice. Still, he remained uncomfortable. The plan was a Hail Mary: an immunotherapy drug, offered in hopes of easing his pain. His wife stared straight into my eyes, holding on to the belief that this medicine would save him.

"When will he start feeling better after the medicine?"

I took a minute, trying to see it the way she did.

"This medicine usually takes a few weeks to work."

Her eyes widened, as if hearing it for the first time.

Frank looked like he had days, not weeks.

I glanced toward my computer. The cursor blinked, the room heavy with grief and hope.

His daughter stood, looking at Frank, then at me, then back at him. A silence settled—heavy, necessary. She took a breath, steadying herself.

"Dad, do you want to be more comfortable? Or do you want to get this drug and keep coming here every three weeks?"

"I just want to be comfortable," Frank whispered, his voice shaking, the words draining what little strength he had left. His eyes closed again.

His labs came back: kidney failure. He didn't qualify for treatment that day.

"I'll talk to the provider and get Palliative to come speak with you both," I told his daughter. She nodded, working her throat as if trying to speak. I offered a hug, and she embraced it.

Palliative came chairside immediately.

He was moved to the bedroom, given more pain medication, and home hospice was arranged.

When I re-entered the room, Frank lay more comfortably, his breathing steadier. The tension had softened.

As hospice placed him onto the stretcher, his daughter turned to me.

"Thank you for everything you do. You're in the right place."

Tears welled in my eyes, burning at the edges.

"Thank you," I managed.

I didn't do anything remarkable. I simply stood in the space between hope and reality—the place oncology nurses often live.

DR. SMALLS

Every three weeks, a new scan. A new doctor. A new set of questions.

I only saw Dr. Smalls once. The high-risk clinic had an abundance of specialists, so I rarely saw the same doctor twice.

He treated us like a task to complete, not people to understand. Busy eyes, curt tone, posture pulled tight.

"Mrs. Wedmore," he said as the door clicked shut.

"Yes." My heart was racing.

"Something is going on with these babies; we don't know what."

I raised my eyebrows.

"What do you mean?"

"Well, Baby A is growing fine. The other is growing, but he's small." He took a sip of his water, scanning me from head to toe. "You aren't small. Any small family members?" he asked, as if genetics were the only lens worth looking through.

My pulse thudded in my ears.

"But the babies are identical?" I pointed out.

"Yes, well . . ." He shrugged. "He's likely not going to be a basketball player," he said, dismissing my concern. I glanced at Dave. His jaw tightened.

"So, just to clarify, our biggest concern today is Baby B's sports career?"

Dr. Smalls registered my displeasure. "Mrs. Wedmore, we really don't know why there is such a difference in the babies' growth."

Science can map genes and predict loss, but every scan still brings more questions—some real, some noise, some only time can interpret. Blending medicine with meaning requires a tolerance for uncertainty. And Dr. Smalls, it seemed, had no patience for the questions that don't come with answers. Maybe he was tired. Maybe he'd seen too much. But I needed more.

I left the appointment oddly reassured—if only because the worst thing he could name was a future without basketball.

TAKE WHAT YOU NEED

"Here's my email—reach out anytime." Siena pressed a folded Post-it into my hand.

"Twins are a gift. You're lucky."

She looked up from her journal, her eyes meeting mine. Something in me eased.

"I had a lot of worries with my second set of twins. It's hard to hear the doctors' concerns and remember they're just doing their job."

She paused, glancing at her chemotherapy bag. The faint hum of the IV pump filled the silence. "But you have to let go of what doesn't serve you."

I nodded. Since early pregnancy, I'd been living scan to scan, worry to worry.

"I do that with this," she said, gesturing to the IV. "My prognosis was always curative, but there's a lot my doctors don't account for." Her steady voice carried an undercurrent of vulnerability.

"Like what?" I asked, almost without thinking. I was on autopilot—teaching chemotherapy, rarely questioning anything beyond the protocol.

"Like preserving my well-being. Hormones. Skin after radiation. Energy. Adrenals after steroids. Things no one prepares you for."

Heat crept up my neck. I hadn't even considered those questions. I hadn't thought past the treatment. Not once.

"Yes, our focus is solely on killing the cancer," I muttered.

Siena slid her pen into her journal sleeve, eyeing me like she'd stumbled upon a teaching moment. "I'm grateful. But still —soda and cookies are served here with lunch?" We laughed, the absurdity hanging in the air.

"We don't treat the cause. We just keep the routine."

Siena nodded, a pause of recognition passing between us.

"This integrative oncology program is a start," she said, "but it's still lacking. I'm doing everything on my own—no guidance on diet, hormones, supplements. Just cancer treatment."

I exhaled, feeling how tightly I'd been holding everything—both at work and in my body.

"Take what you need from the doctors and leave what doesn't serve you," Siena said. "Trust the evolutionary process." Her glacier-blue eyes held steady as she stretched, crossing her long legs. Her gaze held mine. "Like a mother's intuition."

Siena was my New Teach, but she wasn't learning. And I wasn't teaching.

She was reminding me of what I'd pushed aside.

Instinct. Resilience. The quiet things you know before anyone names them.

34.5 WEEKS

When Dr. T. walked through the door, a wave of fear coursed through me. I remembered the way her gaze had terrified me the first time we met. Her presence was still commanding, but her eyes held something different this time. Something softer. Maybe hope.

"Hello, Tara."

"I remember you," I said, suddenly aware of how many versions of me had sat in that chair.

"You got these boys to 34.5 weeks; well done."

I held onto the word done.

Dr. T. eased her stool toward my bed, uncomfortably close. Her tone softened, threading something personal into the clinical.

"If you were my sister, I'd tell you to deliver these babies today."

I nodded, doubt pressed against my ribs like a second heartbeat.

"Can we wait till Monday? See if it's improved?" It was Friday. The ultrasound showed backflow on Baby B's umbilical cord.

She shook her head. “Mono-di twins are high risk. I strongly advise delivery today.”

I let out a long sigh. “Okay.”

She added with a smile, “It’s time for some birthdays.”

“Still ski season too,” Dave said with a laugh.

Dr. T. exited the room.

She would not be the one delivering my boys—it was a Friday evening, and her shift was ending.

Three years later, to the day, I’d run into her once more on a playground, my boys zipping around her and her children like pups let loose.

JUST THE THREE OF US

The boys entered the world at 3.15 and 5.11 lbs. Our greeting was brief, lost between anesthesia and the curtain that separated us. Dave snagged a photo, but all I saw was a blur of blue. The nurses whisked them off to the NICU before I could even hear a cry. The anesthesia haze didn't dull the fear pressing against my chest.

Are they okay?

Why didn't I hear them crying?

"They cried," Dave said gently. "You just missed it."

I felt like I was already missing it all.

Dave wheeled me toward the NICU as soon as I was allowed. My heart rushed with trepidation. Baby A was on the left, the bigger baby, lying peacefully in his cocoon blanket, swallowed by the glass incubator. Baby B was on my right, just as strong but tangled in tubes—feeding, monitoring, transitioning him into the world. Tears welled as I imagined breaking through the glass and pulling them toward me. But all I could do was watch. Tubes replaced me, filling the space I couldn't reach.

Nausea crept in fast, mingling with the ache in my heart.

Could they survive without this place? Would we, the three of us, have been fine on our own?

I reached into each incubator, extending my arms into a T, placing a finger in each tiny hand. Tiny fingers wrapped tightly around mine. Just the three of us, holding on in the only way we could.

SEVENTEEN DAYS

The nurses carried the babies like stardust. They celebrated every gram gained—the first latch, the first full bottle, their tiny hands reunited.

The monitors blinked, pulsed, chimed. Heart rates, oxygen levels—tiny fluctuations that carried so much meaning.

I learned quickly the language of preemies: their cries, their cues, their sheer exhaustion after a few moments at the breast.

"They're not supposed to be here yet," the nurses would remind me when defeat painted my face.

I held them skin-to-skin. Their fingers clung to mine.

The doctors kept saying, "One day at a time. They have to take all their feeds before they can go home."

In the NICU, I missed Addy. At home, I missed the boys.

Dave held each baby on his forearm, lifting them toward his words. "We'll climb more mountains than this," he said.

"They're ready," the doctor announced one morning, smiling without warning. "They both took all their feeds. Simultaneously."

He lingered on the word simultaneously, like it meant more than nutrition.

"Identical twins can be on the same page like that," he said.

The nurse added, flat and certain, "They're going to rock your world."

It didn't feel like encouragement. It felt like a dare.

I smiled anyway.

Seventeen days after they entered the world, they had already taught us resilience—the kind that defies odds, blooms in glass boxes, and echoes through bone.

A MOTHER'S LOVE

I didn't realize how much I needed my mother until I became one. My world felt rocked—the nurse was right, even though I didn't want her to be. My mom folded herself into our chaos like she'd always belonged there. Diapering, rocking, doing 4 a.m. feeds. Holding space, holding babies, holding me.

With the boys home and Addy toddling around, she became a steady presence in a whirlwind of need.

She was there when we needed her most—and when I didn't even know we needed her.

She was there at my noon wedding without ID, and no one dared tell her otherwise.

She's the kind of mother who says yes before you even ask. What I didn't realize then—but know now—is that she taught me how to show up. How to make love a verb.

Her presence rooted me—not to hold me back, but so I could lift my children without losing myself.

THE PERFECT STORM

I wasn't writing much—I was wiping tears, holding bottles, forgetting what day it was.

My visions of a peaceful stroller walk dissolved into cries, spring air nipping at my leaky breasts. I reheated my coffee three times before I drank it. Sleep came in clips. The days blurred—a loop of need and motion.

I counted down the hours until the next stretch of sleep, my voice thinning with each lullaby. "This is hard," I admitted, guilt gnawing at me. "I'm complaining about the babies I prayed so hard for."

"You can love them and need a break," Siena reminded me in one of her many supportive emails. "This is hard on everyone. Give your babies—and yourself—some grace."

I reread Siena's message more than once, clinging to her words like something that could keep me afloat.

Strangers smiled and said, "It goes fast."

My days stayed long.

Somewhere between boredom and exhaustion, I reached out to Meg, sending her a photo of Addison kneeling to feed the boys, both tucked into their Boppys like tiny passengers. My phone immediately rang. It was Meg.

"Delegating—I like it. What do you need? Other than a third arm?"

I laughed for the first time that day.

"Sleep," I said. "And definitely a clone."

"You've got this," she said with a chuckle. "At least…Addy's feeding the boys. That's leadership potential."

"At least I'm not lonely," I added, leaning into the rhythm of the game. I loved it—equal parts comedy and coping mechanism.

Rocky's head rested on my lap, steady. I ran my fingers through his fur, trying to stay tethered as the cries picked up. Addy was asking me something I couldn't quite understand.

"At least you don't have a third arm," Meg said. "That'd look weird in family photos."

We laughed. The game didn't fix anything, but it shifted my perspective—like how one patient's story can reframe a whole day.

Meg stayed on the line long enough for me to remember who I was beyond motherhood. When we hung up, I held them close, all three at once. When the world spun too fast, I moved at their pace. Slowly, it felt less like an impossible climb and more like a storm rearranging my universe.

Walking back into the hospital after maternity leave felt like stepping into a different version of myself. Chaos followed me everywhere, but work was a storm with adults and conversation.

I went back not because life was calmer but because my patients reminded me how to breathe inside the chaos. UPMC had upgraded the facility while I was gone—the rooms sleek and serene, soft tan walls framing nature scenes. Even the nurse' station felt brighter. And so did the nurses. An Integrative

Oncology Center was now on our floor—yoga, mindfulness, massage. Work didn't erase the chaos, but it gave me a foothold.

VISION

Time felt like a carnival mirror, bent and whole at once. Motherhood stretched me between presence and longing, stillness and motion. Then Dolly's voice broke through, grounding me with a wisdom that held both.

"Well hello there, Tara," she said, lifting her head before I spoke. "I'd know that laugh anywhere—it's lighter than the others. And your stride is longer. I can hear it."

She smiled, arms drifting toward me like we were playing Marco Polo. "Walk me to the bathroom?" she asked, reaching for my arm the way my grandmother once did.

She held tight as I led her down the hall, her voice rising into song. She drifted into *Somewhere Over the Rainbow*, her voice thin but sure.

I smiled at the door. "Would you like me to come in?"

She teased, "Oh, I need you, honey—I've got nothing to hide."

We chuckled as I guided her in.

In her seventies, Dolly moved through the world attuned to its quiet rhythms; born blind, listening was a kind of second skin. She knew nurses by the cadence of their steps and the timbre of their laugh, and she often drifted into song.

"All set, Tara," she said as I guided her from the bathroom. As we walked back to her room, she picked up the melody again, unprompted.

Her voice floated through the hallway, tender and cracked. I wondered how she could sing about a world she had never seen, and whether sight had anything to do with sensing beauty the way she did.

"Dolly, your voice is beautiful."

She turned her head toward me, eyes lifting as if reaching for a memory tucked somewhere deep. "I sing of a world I feel."

I smiled, unsure if she could sense it. "Are you always this present?"

"You smile a lot," she said, settling into her treatment chair with a soft thud. "I can hear it. You see, Miss Tara, I can't watch TV or stare at a phone," she said, then chuckled—a laugh that kept going. "But I can still hear and feel. I go to operas and comedians, symphonies and concerts."

Her world was tuned differently. It felt more alive. I couldn't remember when I'd stopped noticing the world that way.

She paused and reached for my hand. "Well, we all start out with awe," she said, squeezing my hand as if she could touch my soul. "Tara, do you remember putting your face against your grandmother's face?"

I did. The memory surfaced: standing atop her long stairwell, saying goodbye, my young face pressed to her soft, wrinkled cheek. Over thirty years ago, still clear as day.

"I do."

"That was a feeling. My sight is made of feelings." She paused. "Children are like that, too. They explore the world with all their senses."

I sighed, fumbling for my curiosity. "I wish I hadn't lost that."

"Oh, Tara, you didn't," she said gently. "Some days I don't

sense beauty either. I envy those who can see the flowers I can only smell, and on those days, I'm just getting by. But when we stop noticing the world around us, time slips away."

"Yes," I admitted. "Some days I'm just waiting for bedtime."

"Oh well," she said, laughing, her eyelids closing with song. "Some days we are so damned tired!"

Her laughter mixed with mine as she softened into melody.

She drifted into that Louis Armstrong classic about trees of green and babies growing.

I thought about my own babies at home, and all the moments slipping through the cracks of chaos and exhaustion.

Maybe Dolly saw more than I did.

REMISSION

I exhaled as the kids went down for naps. The living room stilled after the morning run-around. I opened Siena's email, protein bar in hand.

Siena and I emailed often. She shared tips on feeding and nap schedules, and suggested we take the dogs on hikes for a breather.

"Tara, it's a different battle now," she wrote. "I have to settle my mind in new ways. Otherwise, recurrence wears on the spirit."

The mental gymnastics of remission—a terrain I'd never walked.

I glanced at the monitor, watching my babies' chests rise and fall. I stared at the screen, searching for words. How do I relate?

Siena followed the recommended scans for remission. But she wanted more. She met with a functional medicine doctor. She sought testing beyond standard bloodwork, searching for overlooked imbalances. The more I learned, the more I questioned my own path and what I was missing. I kept reading, feeling something move inside me.

"I try to be grateful—it helps the self-chatter," she wrote. "But we hit another hurdle."

I was loading my old workout DVD when I read Siena's last line.

"Caleb has cancer."

The DVD slipped from my hands and shattered. My fingers trembled. Her husband's cancer was everywhere.

GETTING LOUDER

I wasn't there for a patient. I was there for Siena's husband.

Just months earlier, I'd watched her fight. He sat in the chair beside her. They told me about their children, their parenting tips, the dogs they rescued. And now he was here too. Same chairs. Different floor. Same look: resolute, exhausted.

When I walked into the room, Caleb was sitting tall on the edge of the bed, back straight, shoulders square. Feet pressed firm, as if ready to leap forward, not fall back. He looked too good—healthy, whole. Somehow, that made it worse.

How does this happen twice in one young family?

His eyes met mine.

"I have a lot of life left in me, Tara," he said, steady-eyed.

I nodded. And then I listened, because that's all I had.

He talked about mindset, prayer, food, and the power of the body to reroute its own fate. He smiled a little.

"I'll be praying for you, Caleb. Stay strong," I told him when I stood to leave.

"I will, thank you for stopping by," he said. His legs remained planted on the floor like he had no intention of staying in that bed.

I walked down the hallway and lingered in the atrium before returning to my floor. Sunlight fractured through the glass ceiling. Everything looked the same. But something in me woke up.

Is something in our world making us sick—and why aren't we talking about it?

What does it mean that I'm seeing this more and more? Young patients, same household, same year.

This wasn't a coincidence I could wave away with risk factors or vague theories. There was no box for this in our charting system. No diagnosis code for "what the hell is happening to our environment."

I spent years treating cancer. Now, I was wondering what we were all swimming in while we smiled politely through the slow unraveling.

I didn't have answers. But the questions were getting louder.

STAYING AWAKE

There was just a feeling. A quiet unease. A sense that something in our homes was betraying us.

I sat on the porch, legs tucked beneath me, the baby monitor humming beside a half-drunk glass of wine. The air smelled faintly of citronella and leftover dinner. Dave and I were supposed to be connecting, but I was struggling to stay awake.

My phone buzzed with questions from friends who were waking up alongside me.

Shannon: "Where do I even begin?"

Meg: "Do I really need to spend $30 on beeswax paper? Is tinfoil really that bad?"

I laughed because I felt the same. I told Shannon, "One product at a time." To Meg: "I didn't even know tinfoil was bad?" Both sent the same wide-eyed, overwhelmed emoji face.

I looked down at my hands, still faintly scented from the lavender dish soap I'd just swapped in. "You know what's wild?" I said to Dave, reaching for my glass of wine. "I've spent years working in oncology—educating patients about hormone-sensitive drugs—and I was still using deodorant filled with crap. Every day."

Dave raised his eyebrows. He went along with my swapping out products and meals, always surprised by the latest information I threw at him.

"It's normal to just trust the shelves," he said.

I blinked hard, tiredness settling behind my eyes. "True. I guess we don't question what feels normal. Until it doesn't."

I'd been messaging Siena, knowing she had been making changes long before I did. What do you use for cleaning spray? What about makeup? Do you have a list of trusted sites? She wrote back quickly: "EWG for product ratings. Reverse osmosis filter."

Then came the links. Screenshots. Product reviews.

I wasn't revamping much. I was just beginning to ask questions.

I'd guided patients through hormone-sensitive cancers for years, yet I never mentioned endocrine disruptors. Not because I didn't care. Because it wasn't part of the education. Because I didn't know.

We treat the symptoms. We rarely ask about the cause.

I didn't know my deodorant carried parabens, my shampoo phthalates, my baby wipes synthetic fragrance.

I trusted the water my toddlers drank, unaware of PFAS, pharmaceutical residues, and runoff slipping past municipal tests. I didn't know what I was bringing into my home, onto my body, into my children's lives.

And I was learning.

It was a chapter of beginning—of swapping links with friends who were waking up alongside me. Of reading labels like they were clues. Of asking questions I hadn't known to ask.

We weren't trying to control the uncontrollable. We were trying to live with intention in a world that rarely made it easy. And somehow, that felt like enough. For now.

I leaned back into the porch cushion, the baby monitor still humming, the citronella fading into the night. Dave reached for his empty glass and clinked it gently against mine.

"Hey," he said, his voice low and steady. "You're doing the best you can with what you know."

I smiled, tired and grateful. We raised our glasses anyway. Cheers to staying awake.

LITTLE BLUE BOOK

"I don't want to die, Tara." Carl's words jolted me back to the present. Wrinkles lined his face, and weariness pulled at his gaze. He looked like a man dropped into the ocean without knowing how to swim.

"I still have a lot of life in me."

At seventy-two, he carried a weight you could feel even in a first meeting. I held the binder of chemotherapy side effects—standard for a first visit. But Carl wasn't in a place for standard. He needed conversation, not protocol. I made a mental note to loop in palliative care; they were better at sitting with fear than any binder ever could be.

"Okay, we can talk about that," I said, pulling up a chair beside him and placing the binder on my lap.

Some patients hear only half of what the doctors say. After a gauntlet of tests and appointments, the word "cancer" lands, and everything else blurs. The treatment room becomes the place where it all spills out. Carl sat alone in his big room, a little blue book open on his lap.

"I am dying, right?" His voice trembled beneath the volume.

I told Carl what he already knew. "Well, the hope is this chemotherapy does its job and keeps you alive."

"But if it doesn't do its job, I'm going to die."

He wasn't wrong. Some tumors don't respond to treatment. When cancer keeps growing, it spreads into the places the healthy cells once lived.

"Yes."

"I'm not ready to die. It's terrifying to think about, you know?" he shouted—his everyday volume, I was learning.

I tried to reassure him again, but he spoke over me.

"This is much different than just getting hit by a car. This makes you think, you know? It's the unknown of it."

Carl was already living in the what-ifs. His plan was aggressive chemo, with hope of shrinking the tumor into something manageable. A chronic disease. His prognosis was promising, but it meant treatment for the long haul.

"Ever since this diagnosis, I've been thinking about death," he said again.

"Tell me about your life, Carl. Who will support you through this?" I asked, sensing that I was it.

He frowned. "No one, Tara. I am going to die alone. Do you know how scary that is?"

I felt the truth of it settle between us.

He started talking about his childhood—the yelling, the slammed doors, parents who hated each other, the brother he hadn't spoken to in forty-five years. He'd left their Philly apartment at eighteen and never went back, not even for the funerals.

"It's amazing how much our childhood shapes us," he said, the lines on his face deepening as he spoke. "Do you have any children, Tara?" he asked, pulling me out of my thoughts.

I rarely talked about my kids at work, but people often wanted to know the life behind the scrubs. I let him in a bit and told him about my three. His smile widened—he wanted to know everything.

"See, I can tell your kids adore you because you've shown you care about an old miserable grump like me. I'm sure your kids are much cuter than me too," he chuckled.

"And just as loud," I said.

We laughed as he opened his little blue book.

"So, the side effects, Carl," I said as his hand moved quickly across the page. I paused, realizing he wasn't with me anymore. "I'll be back in a few, Carl."

He didn't look up. He was too deep in whatever he was writing.

DARK HOLLOW

I was supposed to be seasoned in unexpected loss. But I wasn't convinced preparing for death ever worked that way—if the reminders that it can happen at any time made me more vulnerable or less.

"Call me," read the text from my dad. "It's Rocky."

My stomach knotted. Rocky had been sluggish the past few weeks, but it was ninety-five degrees and heavy. I grabbed my phone and stepped into a quiet corner. I was working my one shift that week. My dad had taken Rocky to his place in New Jersey for a week. I'd gratefully accepted the help.

"I'll be right back," I whispered to a coworker, afraid to explain what I didn't want to hear.

The dial tone felt endless, each ring amplifying the wait.

"Hey—I'm at the vet with Rocky," my dad said, his voice heavy. "He couldn't move this morning. They did a scan. Cancer's everywhere."

My hands trembled. Tears soaked my scrub top. Rocky was my Velcro dog. I'd rescued him ten years ago—ten years ago to the month.

"I'm coming home."

"That's too much for you," my dad said gently. "You have babies at home who need you. I can be with him."

His words made me ache for the loss Rocky had already felt —going from all my love to sharing me with four other beings. I hadn't realized there was that much room in my heart. Maybe Rocky hadn't either.

"I need to be there for him."

"Well, if you have to," my dad said, knowing he couldn't hold me back.

I returned to work in a blur. Grief hit fast and hard, erasing my ability to focus. "My dog is dying. I need to be with him," I managed to say.

"I'm so sorry, Tara," my manager said. "Do what you need to do. We'll be fine here."

I reached my car before the phone rang again.

"He's gone," my dad said, emotional now too. "I walked back into the room—he was gone. He decided for you."

He died alone. My chest felt heavy. I muttered between sobs, "Thank you, Dad," as I drove to the one place I thought I could find solace: Dark Hollow.

I scaled the cliffside, grief clinging with heavy breath and tears. My heart ached for him.

I stopped at the ascent. Dark Hollow looked different, like a place I didn't want to explore without my explorer. Oak trees blocked the sky, their canopy shading the heat. Sweat and tears burned my eyes. Rocky was always right there when I cried, pressing his soft black fur into my legs, my arms—my heart.

The stream ran below, winding through the valley toward a small trickling waterfall. I remembered our first trip there years earlier—his effortless descent, his beeline for the water. The slow trickle was the same that day. Water shapes rock over time. Loss had shaped me too.

There was a time when I didn't think anyone—or any creature—needed me. My walls were high, my defenses strong, like

Rocky in that kennel cage. But as I stood beside the waterfall, I understood something simple: he didn't just need me. We needed each other.

"We love you, Rocky!" I shouted into the valley. "Now run free like you always do," I whispered. "I will be forever grateful for meeting your wild soul," my voice echoed off the mountainside.

I sat on a boulder beneath my trembling legs. And I prayed. I prayed that all our adventures and all the love I gave him covered the one time I wasn't there.

Maybe he was trying to teach me that love doesn't always need a final moment. It just needs to be lived well enough to let go.

THE FLOOR ABOVE

I always tried to stop in when Caleb was there. It was one of those days when the to-do list barely left room to breathe. But a rare lull in my schedule gave me just enough time to slip upstairs, to the floor where he was receiving his infusion.

The layout was different—less familiar. I scanned the room and found him propped up in the recliner, a blanket tucked neatly at his waist. And beside him, Siena.

She looked up as I approached, her smile the kind that had weathered things—grief, hope, uncertainty.

"You didn't have to come," she said. Her voice was soft but certain, like she already knew the answer.

"I know," I replied, sliding into the empty chair. "But I wanted to."

Caleb gave me a nod, his signature quiet strength still intact. There were dark moons under his eyes, but his posture—upright, steady—was the same as the first day I met him. Feet planted. Refusing to sink.

We talked for a while—not about side effects or scans—but about their kids, softball, Siena's latest attempt at sourdough. It felt like stealing sunlight during a storm.

When Caleb dozed off, Siena leaned back and stared at the IV line. "You know," she said, "I used to think the worst thing was being sick. But sitting here . . ." She trailed off, then looked at me. "This side's harder, in some ways. Watching. Waiting."

I met her gaze and stayed there, steady—the way she once did for me in a cramped room when I couldn't find the words for my own fear.

We sat like that for a while, two people who've both been on either side of the chair, in our own way.

Some friendships don't need a thousand texts or perfectly timed visits.

WHAT HE SAID IN THE RAIN

Addison and I stopped for a quick bite on a steamy August morning. I didn't notice the tall figure leaning against the half-wall until his familiar toothpick smile caught my eye.

"Hey, you," he said.

"Jack!" I shouted, shooting upward, open-armed. Seeing patients outside the hospital always felt like catching a glimpse of life stealing a victory lap.

"I got the dogs in the truck. Come meet them," he insisted, making goofy faces at Addy as we walked beside him. She giggled.

"You look great, Jack."

"Feeling great, too—scans are still clear."

Outside, the clouds pressed low. His German shepherds hung their stoic heads from the pickup, tails wagging as Addy squealed at their generous licks.

"Jack, I better get going. I rode my bike," I said, pointing toward the dark sky.

"Hop in, I'll give you a lift."

"It's okay, we can get home quick." I didn't want to impose—or maybe I wasn't ready to be seen outside the roles we knew.

"Suit yourself," Jack said with his trademark wink.

I pedaled hard as the rain fell sharp and fast. Jack's blue pickup surged forward through the blur, his lips moving in words I couldn't catch. He waved, then vanished into the gray curtain.

A couple months later, I learned Jack had died unexpectedly —still cancer-free. The news hit with the kind of shock you never get used to. I replayed that rainy morning again and again, wishing I'd stretched it longer, wishing I'd caught whatever he was trying to say.

Life is full of almosts and unanswered questions, threads we carry and untangle in time. Some goodbyes last because you didn't know they were happening.

AN ACQUIRED TASTE

"I want Tara! Is Tara here today? Tara, I want Tara!"

He was shouting at the secretary from a foot away, unaware of how loud he was or how many people were wincing. He reminded me of my toddlers—loud, persistent, unconcerned with social norms. But Carl was a grown man, and the waiting room's annoyance was palpable. I chuckled and waved from down the hall.

Carl was an acquired taste. Most nurses found him brash; I welcomed him. He liked familiarity and our budding friendship. Most days, I did too. He was responding well to chemotherapy —the tumor was shrinking as hoped.

Carl launched into a tangent about his side effects. "I enjoy talking to you, Tara," he said, then barreled on before I could answer. "As a dying man, I can say whatever I feel now."

"Can you really, Carl?"

I had a hard time believing he was ever any different. Carl spoke in run-ons, like he feared someone might cut him off before he finished.

He chuckled. "I'm a glassblower. I work in my basement alone; I do better that way." He paused, contemplative. "But I think it gave me this lung cancer; protective gear wasn't a thing in the past. My ex-girlfriend always told me to cover my face, but I never listened. Maggie…have I told you about Maggie?"

"No."

"We dated for thirty-five years. We never married—she wanted marriage. She wound up marrying some other guy."

I didn't know what to say, so I said nothing.

"She's actually my ride today—oh, you'll have to call her when I'm done; I don't have a cell phone."

He pulled a crumpled piece of paper from his blue book, numbers scribbled across it in shaky ink.

"Sure," I said, grateful for the task and a break in his monologue.

Maggie answered like she'd been waiting by the phone all morning, her voice warm and ready. She arrived within minutes, arms full of snacks. Carl dismissed them immediately.

"I just had chemotherapy. Why would you think I'd want snacks!"

She tucked them back into her purse, dropping some along the way. I bent to help her pick one up. As they exited, his voice rose again, sharp with an anger I couldn't place.

TO THE BOYS

Erin flashed her red lipstick-lined smile as she adjusted her wig like a bike helmet, then reached for my arm to steady herself as she rose from the wheelchair. Erin was my age, and I loved seeing her as much as she unsettled me—a reminder that cancer can and does happen to someone just like me.

She'd been diagnosed young with metastatic breast cancer and was now on salvage treatment.

"Good to see you again," Erin said. "My legs are sore." She paused to catch her breath. "My husband and I just spent the weekend in nature, hiking."

"That sounds so nice." I wondered how she'd hiked yesterday as I tucked warm blanket after warm blanket around her shrinking frame.

"I couldn't really hike far," she said, answering the question I hadn't asked. "And we left the boys with my parents. They would have loved it."

Her words carried a trace of regret—the kind that lingers when time with loved ones slips away. I felt it echo in me as I wrestled with the same balance, trying to stretch myself across those I love. Erin felt it too; her urgency was visible, but mine was no less real.

I steadied my voice. "That sounds lovely, Erin. What a beautiful weekend for it. Was the fall foliage nice?"

But Erin wasn't into small talk anymore.

"I wrote to my boys about it and told them the spots I loved. We're going back on Christmas and hopefully it'll snow. It's really pretty there with snow."

My expression shifted before I could hide it. She *wrote* to them?

"Oh, I thought I told you. I made email accounts for the kids. I send them little stories—things that happened with us, ideas I have, and every birthday I write about that version of themselves."

Her words hung in the air. Erin was writing herself into the future for her children.

Her kids were the same ages as mine.

"I'm not sure how much time I have," she said. "I want my kids to know me—and us—through me. Not just through pictures or other people's memories. And hopefully, they'll have some real ones of their own."

"That's such a beautiful idea. May I borrow it?"

Her smile grew with excitement.

"Of course! It's yours to borrow. I plan to give it to them when they enter adulthood if I'm still here; otherwise, I hope my husband will know when the time feels right."

She sighed.

My eyes welled some more, filling the space where words should have been.

The silence stretched. I wanted to sit with it, to offer something meaningful, but all I could do was nod. I retreated to the one thing I knew—her treatment plan.

A WHITE ONE

Her disease had been advancing. I knew that. But the change still stunned me; even when you expect it, the body's unraveling always feels abrupt.

We were at a crowded city-lights Christmas event with the family—the kind of place you don't expect to see a patient, which is why it felt like life was handing me a final moment with her. As I shouldered through the chaos, trying to keep my eyes on my three, I bumped into a wheelchair.

I nearly landed in her lap.

Erin.

She wore her brunette wig, blankets over jackets, layers upon layers. She was smaller than I remembered.

"Hi Erin," I said, my tone and face carrying what my words couldn't as I leaned in for a hug. There was a flicker of recognition, but she seemed far away. As her kids zigzagged around the wheelchair, a small smile appeared.

My three darted off, and I followed. We exchanged only a few words, but I trusted the meaning of our encounter.

Erin passed away a couple days after Christmas. It was a white one.

I think of Erin often—usually when I write to my children. The stories I send them aren't glamorous. They are fragments of now, stitched together so they'll know me in ways photographs can't. Erin taught me that love can be written forward.

THE CLIMB

I clipped into the Peloton, my anchor of consistency as we exited the holiday chaos. The house was quiet, still humming from Christmas, the kids still asleep. I was tired in that way sleep can't fix. But I chose movement.

Exercise has always been my medicine. Where I process. Where I remember.

Sweat gathered quickly. My mind drifted—to Cooper asking to be held again, and the quiet ache that followed: one day, I won't be holding you. To Addison wondering if Rocky was chasing squirrels in heaven. The questions that catch me off guard. The ones that stay.

"You woke up today," the instructor shouted, electric. "Do you know how lucky you are?!"

The words landed in my chest. I woke up. I moved. I felt.

Every day, I witness people who would give anything to feel their heart pounding from effort instead of fear. Maya used to hike every Friday. "I miss the sun on my face," she told me once. "I miss the way it made me feel like myself."

And still, they showed up. They smiled. They found joy in the smallest movements.

I turned the resistance knob and climbed. The grief. The gratitude. The ache of watching my children grow and the privilege of being able to witness.

I've cried on this bike. I've laughed. I've prayed.

It's not just a workout. It's where I return to myself. Where I remember I'm still here. Still moving.

I turned the knob to the right. My legs burned. My breath caught. And still, I climbed.

Because I could.

THE VIRUS

"The scan was stable, which means: still dying, just not today," he said with a smirk as he looked out the window. I adjusted the IV volume, unsure how to respond. The television played a loop about "a virus spreading overseas." Nurses were talking about it at the station too. No answers, just circle talking.

"You think this thing's serious? The virus?" He wasn't panicked. Just curious. A man who'd already faced things scarier than breaking news.

"They say it's still overseas," I offered, somewhere between professional calm and personal uncertainty.

"Eh. I'm not worried about it."

I glanced at him. No bitterness. No drama. Just truth. Like someone commenting on the weather.

That's the thing about patients at the edge: the ones closest to death often seem the least afraid of it.

Outside, the hallway felt like a weather pattern shifting. You could sense it in the way coworkers lingered over updates and how sanitizer bottles sprouted everywhere—bright, out of place, necessary.

MAUREEN'S TRAIL

We departed for Big Sky with change in the air. We were on the brink of a pandemic, but the mountains were calling. I hugged my children goodbye and felt like I was losing a limb. They did, too. As toddlers, they didn't understand why I needed the mountains at all.

We traveled with friends who had also left their kids with grandparents. As hard as parting was, it felt freeing to ski without responsibilities. But the sky told a different story. Even the clouds looked foreboding as we ascended toward Big Sky.

It was a powder day. The firs and aspens were dusted like flour, white against dark green needles. The sky was as big and beautiful as I remembered, amplified by the foot of snow.

"My meeting is at noon," our friend said, disappointed.

"Can't you just tell them it's a powder day?" I asked immediately.

We were on the chairlift, heading out for our first run. The snow was piling up, and my black jacket filled with white fluff. It was a "free refills" kind of day, the powder replenishing the tracked snow after each run.

"Unfortunately, we need to discuss the pandemic." He paused. "It's official now."

Snowboarding on powder is magical. It feels like floating—the body works tirelessly, but the exertion is easy to miss. The sheer pleasure takes over: turning, flying, soaring.

And then the anxiety hit. My phone lit up with mom groups in a frenzy—playgrounds closed, lockdowns looming. My kids felt a planet away.

The sky suddenly looked foreign, the beauty harder to see. The news snapped me out of it, the calm gone in an instant. Dave stayed steady.

"If we have to, we'll rent a car and drive home," he said.

His logic calmed me, but I still missed the kids.

The day was beautiful. A bluebird morning. Maya ran through my mind's eye—she always did on bluebird days. We rode the chairlifts packed shoulder to shoulder.

For lunch, we headed to the mid-mountain lodge. The corridor was lined with people waiting to be seated. Beyond the crowd was a vast room of oak, high ceilings, and natural light. We sat at the bar. The bartender filled beers like he was working a conveyor belt. Perhaps we sensed it was the last hurrah in public for a while.

A couple next to us received an email about their daughters' school shutting down. They ordered more beer. We laughed with them, but the uncertainty sat between us. She hugged me for listening. It would be the last time I hugged a stranger for years.

We walked out of the lodge with six inches of fresh powder and an immediate shift in our mental state. The endorphins rose with the afternoon pileup.

We found ourselves taking laps on one trail, Blackfoot—a black diamond through the glades, mostly un-trafficked and incredibly serene. The trail drops off, resembling a precipice into the abyss, making it hair-raising and freeing, wrapped in one tight little turn.

It's the kind of magic that attracts people of a certain stripe. And on a powder day, there is so much joy in the solitude of it all. I stopped frequently to catch my balance and breath. I leaned back into the mountain behind me. The slope caught me as I rested my legs. I looked up at the snow clouds, unveiling a sliver of the heavens above.

Silence met the falling snow.

I was on Maureen's trail.

BROKEN CLOCKS

March 2020 broke clocks. Hours stretched, days blurred. Fear sped time up; boredom slowed it down.

The airport was nearly empty.

We wore masks I'd pocketed from work, flimsy things that felt more like hope than protection. On the plane, a man kept sneezing. People flinched. Then again. And again. The tension on the flight was louder than the engines. I watched the movie Armstrong. Something about his stillness in space matched how disoriented I was beginning to feel. The sky outside the window was endless and close, and we flew through it like ghosts.

It was midnight when we arrived home. I raced up the stairs. I needed to see them. To touch them. To count heads. The boys rolled like wet noodles, tangled in soft breath and fleece pajamas. Addison woke up. Her hug was hard. She didn't speak, just wrapped herself around me until her little body finally exhaled. I held that moment.

The next day, we were advised to quarantine: stay away from anyone but our nuclear family. We waved goodbye to my parents from the porch. Fear rose up their necks and settled in their eyes. We all wore the same anxious stare—wide and searching.

My mom group texted: "Dark times without playgrounds and friends." Outside the sky hung low and colorless, like it knew something we didn't.

We walked to an empty parking lot near the closed gym and silent restaurant. My kids brought scooters. A wineglass sat on the curb, a faint reminder of a last hurrah.

"Race from the white line to me," I called.

They burst forward, three tiny rockets in rain boots and neon, completely oblivious to any world but theirs.

Then we found the puddles. I convinced myself the magic was there. They didn't need convincing. They laughed. They soaked their pant legs. They didn't care.

Time had broken. The night before, it raced; now it hovered, stretching like elastic in the sky above the lot.

We got home. I looked at the clock. It hadn't really moved.

"Are the clocks broken?"

Dave just raised his coffee and chuckled.

The days were bending, like funhouse glass. Long in some places. Short in others. Nothing was consistent but the shift.

It was the beginning of slowing down. Time wasn't measured by hours anymore—just by the rituals of home.

Covid was good for some things: stillness with the people who mattered most.

The outpatient clinic stayed open. Chemo couldn't wait.

Some nurses questioned if we were essential.

"Oh, we're essential," the pharmacist said, handing over a bin of medications.

Another nurse sighed. "We just want to stay home in our PJs like everyone else."

He raised a brow. "No, you don't. That's not glamorous either."

He was right. At work, I held my breath. At home, I couldn't find one.

Eventually, the mask mandate took effect. We felt a little safer, like lining the battlefield with paper walls.

Sip of coffee. Mask up. Granola bar. Mask up. Eight hours of plastic and coffee breath.

Eventually, I started pulling my mask down at my desk. Not out of rebellion. Just for air.

SIENA

The hallway smelled like Lysol and coffee and something metallic I couldn't name. I had just finished charting when I saw her.

Siena.

She wore Hoka running sneakers and carried a small bag—homemade things, always—tied off with her touch.

"I know you're busy," she said. "I just wanted to drop this off."

"You are so sweet. Thank you, Siena."

She shrugged. "Caleb had an appointment. And you sounded like you could use a boost."

Inside the bag: turmeric drops, energy bites, herbal tea, and a folded note I wouldn't read until hours later in my car, when the world felt especially frayed.

FACETIME

I stood outside the room.

The nurse inside held up a phone. FaceTime was glitching, the audio choppy. But you could still hear the daughter's breath —the kind you take when trying not to sob.

"Hi, Mom," she whispered, waving through the screen, a tremor in her hand. "I love you. I'm right here."

The patient blinked slowly, more breath than body. Oxygen hissing. Hands tucked in blankets that had lost their warmth.

We all pretended it was enough.

Later, I sat at the nurses' station, mask damp from the hours. Someone drank stale coffee.

Outside, the world was arguing about whether the virus was real.

Inside, we were holding screens up to dying mothers.

And everyone was doing their best.

THE SECOND TIME AROUND

Jolene was my first New Teach after the hospital's guest policy changed. No more loved ones at bedside. No more hand-holding at the bell. But Jolene didn't shrink—she expanded.

She entered the room with arms flying, commanding the room without trying.

"Hi, I'm Jolene. I'm ready," she announced, her piercing blue eyes looking through me above her mask.

"I'm Tara," I said.

"Tara," she repeated, reaching to shake my hand before instantly pulling back. "We can't do that anymore, huh?" Her mask slipped when she laughed, flashing a cheekbone, a dimple maybe. Beauty had become a guessing game. She adjusted it again without missing a beat, already asking questions, already filling the room. She didn't shrink from the strangeness of it all.

Jolene had HER2-positive breast cancer—a curable diagnosis with a tough regimen ahead.

"I bet you don't sit still for long," I said, watching the way her body naturally shifted, her fingers drumming lightly on the chair, already restless.

Jolene chuckled. "I like you already." She nodded, then narrowed her eyes in curiosity. "So tell me about yourself, Tara. How are you holding up through all this madness? Any kids at home?"

"Yes, I have three little kids at home—twin boys and a girl. They were in preschool; now they're home, bouncing off the walls."

Her eyebrows shot up, her entire face alive with amusement.

"Oh, you're in the thick of it," she said, shaking her head. "That's survival mode right there."

I laughed, because she had a way of making everything feel lighter.

"Those busy little years make marriage hard work," she said. "A lot falls on the mother. I raised four boys, and sometimes I wanted to punch my husband in the face."

Somehow I could still make out her twisted grin beneath her mask. Marriage became logistics: fitting tiny lives into bigger ones.

"I swear, it's like juggling chainsaws some days," Jolene said, rolling her eyes. "The kids pull you in one direction, the house falls apart in another, and somewhere in the middle, your husband is still there, expecting attention—expecting, well, something."

She sighed, arms wide like she was shedding a skin. I came to talk chemo, but somehow, we were deep in marriage survival tactics.

"But you have to protect it—the marriage. Otherwise, it disappears beneath the piles of laundry, meal planning, and appointments. I used to tell my husband, 'I love you, but I'm barely staying afloat over here.'"

"How did you protect it?"

I could hear the smirk in her voice, exhaling like someone about to confess a hard-earned truth.

"I got a divorce."

I didn't expect that.

I burst into a hard laugh.

"But with my second husband," she continued, still grinning, "I learned."

I nodded. "What did you learn? And also, let me know when you're ready to learn about these drugs." I shifted in my stool and pointed to the packet of chemo education.

"Oh yeah, that cancer thing," she said, and we both laughed, comfortable now.

"Honestly, it's just small things. We have coffee together every morning before the kids wake up. Even if it was ten minutes, it was ours. No interruptions, no chaos—just us."

I watched Jolene's hands—unbothered by the IV, still moving, still restless. I reached for the chemo packet.

"Okay," I said, smiling. "Let's talk about these drugs."

She leaned in, finally still.

"Teach me," she said. "I want to know what I'm up against."

DAKOTA

I was wrapping up my charting when my aunt sent a picture. A sleek black lab mix, eyes dark and uncertain.

Dave surprised me with his excitement. "She looks perfect. See if she's good with kids."

I hesitated. I wasn't sure I could handle one more need, one more being to care for. But something about her—those eyes, that timing—made me trust the alignment more than the doubt.

Dakota was a one-year-old black lab/pointer mix who'd spent weeks chained to a neighbor's fence, forgotten in the yard.

When the woman who rescued her knocked on their door and asked why they didn't care for their dog, they shrugged and handed her over. She took Dakota, knowing she needed more than rescue—she needed a home. And we wanted her.

Bringing her home meant a long car ride to North Carolina. When Dave arrived, she was skittish and unsure, her ribs showing, her frame too thin. But she leaned into us.

Addison had a tennis ball waiting. Dakota didn't like fetch, but she liked the way it smelled. Addison pulled blankets up beside her, hopeful she'd stay in her bed. The boys moved with the quick, clumsy hands of toddlers, but Dakota took it all in stride, absorbing the chaos of love as if she'd been waiting for it.

One afternoon, I took her to Dark Hollow. The fall leaves settled on the trail, a quiet place for trust to be tested.

"Here we go," I whispered, unclipping the leash. Dakota trotted ahead, her body tense with possibility. Then, just as quickly, she turned back, seeking me.

Rocky had done the same once. He had known better than to run.

She fit the hollow space he left.

SUSPENDED

The trail crunched beneath my boots, snow lining the edges in pale morning light. Dakota trotted ahead, ears flicking at every sound. Icicles dangled from the cliff, catching the sun.

I paused, picturing my children's wide-eyed wonder. Their small hands would have reached for the frost.

I wanted both: the quiet of these mornings and the chaos of bedtime. To move my body and still be still. To hold joy without exhaustion.

My phone buzzed. Shannon. I carried it for safety, though most days it felt like a leash. I picked up, surprised to hear my own voice say hello.

We didn't talk long—just long enough to circle something real. I told her how the days blurred, how presence felt slippery. She didn't miss a beat. "That's why I'm always chasing newness," she said. "Novelty slows time. Childhood feels long because it's full of firsts. Even if it's messy."

I could hear her grin, probably halfway through a memory of backpacking somewhere wild and uncomfortable. Shannon always threw herself into new experiences. It wasn't glamorous. But it was awake.

"Even this," she added, "this kind of conversation—it makes the moment feel different."

We said goodbye. I slipped the phone back into my pocket. The icicles caught my attention again. They would eventually melt, dripping silently into the earth below. For now, they remained suspended.

WHILE HE WEPT

I walked into Carl's room. His eyes were tired, hollow above a mask that couldn't hide the strain.

"Tara," he said, voice thin but deliberate. "It's great seeing you."

He paused, then added with a huff, "This Covid though… ridiculous, the world we're living in."

I let him talk. His rant wandered—Covid, politics, loneliness. Then he fell quiet and looked up.

"How do patients with lung cancer die, Tara?" His voice broke at the edge.

I was still working on my own discomfort with death. Nursing school doesn't teach you how to answer questions like that—not really. And I was years beyond training.

"Have you spoken to palliative care?" I asked carefully.

Carl didn't like that answer.

"I talked to palliative care already," he said, his voice cracking just enough to hurt. "But I wanted to talk to you, Tara."

He was asking for something deeper. Something honest. I didn't have an answer he needed.

"It's hard," he whispered. "Thinking about dying. About how it happens, you know?"

I nodded. He kept talking, circling around fear and all the things he wasn't ready to lose.

I didn't say much. He didn't need answers. He just needed to be heard.

The chemo had worn him down. Neuropathy crept into his fingers and toes, making it nearly impossible to work the glass the way he loved. A burn from the bench had rattled him, and his oncologist told him to step back from the one thing that still gave him joy. It's a fragile balance, trying to kill the thing that's killing someone without destroying the parts that keep them alive—the parts that still love, still create, still reach for joy.

"I'm leaving my assets to Maggie," he said, eyes down. "I know that sounds strange."

"No, it doesn't," I said. "She cares about you."

He nodded slowly. "She always has. And I have no one else."

His face crumpled. I wanted to hug him, but we were in the throes of a pandemic.

So, I stayed where I was, hands in my pockets.

While he wept.

LOVE ALWAYS, CARL

The charge nurse called, "You have a visitor."

I turned the corner and saw Maggie, her nerves a live wire.

She reached into her purse and dropped her pen as she rummaged through her bag. I knelt to pick it up.

"Maggie, I'm so sorry for your loss; I would hug you if I could," I said, my words muffled by my mask.

Tears welled in her eyes, and I stood helpless, frozen by a virus that kept connection at arm's length.

She pulled Carl's beaten-up blue notebook from her bag and handed me a folded page tucked inside.

"It doesn't look special, but he wanted you to have it."

She stood there waiting for me to read it.

"Maggie, I don't know if I can read this here."

Her head lowered, her gaze shifting to the ground. I folded back the crumpled paper.

As tears fell into my mask, my eyes scanned Carl's scribbled shorthand:

"Tara—my favorite Hillman nurse—listens.

- 3 children who adore her: Addison, Cooper, and Davey (twins)

– Mask now covers a smile that precedes her

Thank you. Keep listening the way you do.

It's rarer than you think.

Hold onto your loved ones. Love is all you need.

Love Always, Carl."

I tucked Carl's crumpled page into my back pocket. Carl always carried that little blue book—the way the rest of us clutched our phones. That evening, I placed it in my memorabilia box like a dandelion—small and unassuming but capable of carrying something far greater than itself. Then I smiled, thinking about how that grumpy old man made his way into my heart, and into the box where I keep the pieces of my life that still have a pulse.

WHAT I'VE KEPT

I keep my memorabilia box quaint. It's an old, worn cardboard box, one toss away from the recycling bin. I've nearly abandoned it with every move, but then I open it.

Inside are cards from old college and high school teams, Wilmot nurses, Thoracic 9, poetic goodbyes from dear friends, a photo or two of dogs gone to heaven, and my grandmother's smiling face pressed beside my own. Every profound note or object I've been given since I began to find meaning lives there.

It usually begins at a crossroads—a parting of the ways, or a gift.

I wish it didn't work that way, but that's what fills my box.

I only open it on rare occasions, usually when I'm adding something new.

I placed Carl's tinted-blue, folded page atop my grandmother's Polaroid photograph—an unlikely duo sharing space. Her warm smile beside his jagged handwriting—two people who would never cross paths now touching in a cardboard box I can't seem to throw away.

The flyer from the Bali yoga retreat had slipped to the top

again, its corners curled like old dreams. It always felt out of reach, something I wasn't quite ready for.

I picked up the Polaroid photo of my grandmother. She'd been my earliest example of quiet resilience. I remember pressing the shutter on those old cameras, waiting for the small square of film to slide out the front. The image always appeared slowly, starting at the edges and working its way inward. The muted colors always blurred and blended, sharpening with time and light. It felt like watching a life experience unfold—how clarity arrives slowly, how lessons take shape only after exposure.

I held up the photo and thought of the patients who had moved through my life, each one leaving something behind.

Not in grand ways, but in small shifts I didn't always notice at the time.

I slipped the picture back into the box.

KINDERGARTEN

Addison's backpack was almost bigger than she was. Pink, with her name across the top and a zipper that stuck if you pulled too fast. Her shoes lit up when she walked, and her braids swayed with every step toward the classroom door.

She held my hand tight, and I wasn't ready to let it go.

A mask covered her sweet little smile.

We asked so much of children that year—follow rules they didn't understand, stay apart in classrooms built for connection.

And they listened.

I stood there longer than I meant to, watching the door close behind her. The outside felt quiet in a way that wasn't peaceful. Just empty.

I teared up in the car. It felt like a beginning and an ending at the same time. I'm not sure either of us were ready.

The next day, a patient asked me what age kids start kindergarten. He would never see his granddaughter start school.

"Five," I said, and he smiled like he was reaching for a memory he'd once held but wouldn't again.

I thought of Addison's romper dress. Her shoes lighting up.

Her brave little wave. Some days, the weight of what I witness makes me hold my own children tighter. Other days, it makes me let go.

THE FACE WE CAN'T COVER

Some patients stayed with me. Not just their names or diagnoses, but the way they made me feel, like I'd been handed something sacred.

Some stories were soft. Others were harder to hold.

Like Mario.

He had a tumor on his jaw so large it distorted his entire face. It made me realize how impossible it is to look at half a face and imagine the other half. It wasn't just swelling—it was protrusion, a visible mass that pulled his skin taut and made his mouth sit crooked.

People stared. Even in the hospital, where we were supposed to know better, I saw the way eyes lingered—not with cruelty, exactly, but with discomfort. Curiosity. Pity.

He hated being looked at.

He wore a hooded sweatshirt even in July, tugging the fabric forward like it might shield him from the world. We didn't make him wear a mask. Some head-and-neck patients simply couldn't.

That was the thing about head and neck cancers—they were

unignorable. Unlike a tumor tucked deep in the lung or colon, these ones lived on the surface. They changed how a person was seen and heard. How they saw themselves.

His treatment was radiation that burned the inside of his mouth—the bright red and pink skin, the altered speech. Chemotherapy made him nauseated and weak. He lost weight quickly, then stopped eating altogether. The pain was too much. Eventually, a feeding tube was placed, and even that felt like a defeat.

He was quiet most of the time. When a large mass is pressing on your ability to make words, it strips away communication. Many head and neck cancer patients showed up with pen and paper. That's how we talked—if you could call it that. I was used to asking the kind of questions that turn a hospital stay into something more like a place where stories are shared, where meaning finds its way into the margins. But with Mario, it would have been easier to stay quiet.

I think Mario liked that I tried. I asked questions, even when I knew the answers would cost me time. "I'm sorry, I know this is hard for you. We don't have to talk if you'd rather rest."

"All I have here is time. And all I do is rest," he wrote, adding a small smiley face after the words. I found a seat, and we wrote notes in silence. I smiled whenever I could. Every once in a while, he'd try to smile with the side of his face that hurt less to move.

One afternoon, we played tic-tac-toe. He looked up from beneath his hoodie as I slid the scribbled board toward him. His crooked smile, elaborate in its effort, was the closest he could come to saying thank you.

And when he was done, when the fight had drained from him, he didn't need to write it. It was in his eyes. I remember thinking how much effort it must have taken just to look up.

Mario's last Post-it to me had that same smiley face, the one he wished his face could make on its own. But I didn't know him then. I don't remember the exact day he died, but I remember the feeling: the kind of relief that comes when suffering finally ends, mixed with wonder. I wondered who Mario was before the tumor took his face, his voice, and then gave him to me.

LIKE A ROLLER COASTER

After a long day riding roller coasters as a child, I'd lie in bed and still feel like I was moving. My stomach would drop with invisible turns. My body couldn't tell the ride was over.

Driving home from work felt the same way. My mind still raced like I was charting. The day replayed in a scattered loop—what did I miss? Did I forget to document something? In the silence, I could finally hear myself again.

Then the garage door opened. I stayed in the hush as long as I could. Three little squeals. A few barks. The chaos of family crashing into the stillness I hadn't yet reached.

It felt like stepping into a circus—chaotic, bright, alive. But the squeals, the sticky hands, the arms flung around me like they were trying to fold me back into the world.

Even Dakota joined the fray, tail thrashing in joy.

They reminded me of what lived beyond the hospital doors. That love is loud and doesn't wait for rest.

And still, the exhaustion on top of exhaustion was real. I wanted the house to be empty. I wanted a shower. Maybe to cry.

But I thought of Erin. And Maya. And Taylor. And all the people who would give anything to walk into a house like this.

Sometimes we count our blessings. Sometimes we don't.
But either way, they're there.
Alive. Waiting. Hanging on me and squealing.
Grace dressed up as noise.

CAN YOU SIT WITH BOTH?

Siena stood out against the sycamores—confident, two leashes in hand.

"How are you?" she asked, freeing her dogs. "I brought you some homemade granola bars," she said, handing me a small box she'd filled with other thoughtful things.

The winter chill met us as we climbed the icy hills of Pittsburgh's woods. The trail was slick, the trees still and frosted—nothing like the hospital, and everything like a space where I could breathe. Siena and I talked about motherhood, but mostly we leaned into well-being, self-care, and what we were moving toward next. Our words tumbled easily. It was different from other friendships. It was unguarded. True.

"We're moving to Delaware," I said just as my boot caught a patch of ice nestled between a tree root and crusted snow. I lurched, grabbing a low branch to steady myself.

"Oh wow! Why?" Siena asked, eyes wide.

"I don't know. We want something different. Coastal life sounds...like a change."

Her silence stretched a beat too long before she answered with a steely stare.

"I felt that way recently." Her voice softened. "I wanted land. Space. Just...something else. I even found a place an hour away that felt like it might give me that. But it didn't sit right. I let it go. Then a year later, something opened up right across the street."

We descended the ridge in silence, the brook humming beside us. Our breath rose in clouds; our boots crunched in rhythm. It felt like the forest was listening.

"Life figured it out for you," I conceded.

"It sure did. But what about you—does Delaware feel right?" Siena asked, her voice low but pointed.

"I'm not sure," I admitted, eyes following the brook's winding path. "Is it ever crystal clear?"

"No," she said. "It takes time. You have to move with it first. Feel the flow."

Her arms pinwheeled briefly to find balance on the slick slope. We both slowed, feet adjusting to the shifting terrain.

"I feel torn," I confessed. "Part of me wants newness—adventure. But another part wants to stay grounded, grow roots."

Siena paused mid-step. "Can you sit with both? Just for a while?"

"I guess so." I didn't explain that if I think too long, I freeze. I've learned that sometimes I need to move first and understand later—like skiing, when hesitating at the edge of a steep, I lose the nerve to drop in.

"Caleb and I live differently now. Cancer changed our perspective. We both have better instincts. But some things don't make sense until you've stood at the edge yourself."

I wondered if some of Siena's perspective—the kind you only get by walking through fire—was starting to rub off on me.

Siena stared off down the slope.

"How are you and Caleb?" I asked. I knew she was in remission, but Caleb's situation had always been more complicated.

She stopped walking.

"Caleb's still under surveillance and on medication, indefinitely. But he's healthy. No detectable cancer." She looked right at me. "And I'm cancer-free." Her words hung like icicles from the eaves, sharp in the cold winter air.

We both knocked on the closest sycamore.

GUARDIAN ANGEL

He handed me a guardian angel pin, picked from a bag full of them.

"You girls are my angels."

I was adjusting his IV tubing, trying not to knock over the cup of ginger ale he liked with crushed ice. It was all he could stomach lately. Dean didn't have many more days left. I hadn't read a note, but he told me without telling me.

He said it so casually, like it was obvious. "You are all angels," he added, nodding weakly.

I smiled, uncomfortable. I didn't feel like an angel. Angels glow. They're serene, divine. I felt tired. Frazzled. My stomach was growling. I had three other patients waiting. My neck hurt. And I needed to pee.

But I'd heard it before—nurses called angels. Maybe that's true for some. But most of us are a mosaic of motion, mess, and grace. Detectives. Mechanics. Listeners. Fixers. Mothers. Mentors. People carrying more than anyone sees.

"Thank you, Dean," I said, tears in my eyes, as I placed the angel pin on my badge—for him to see, for me to carry. His eyes were already closing, but I think he saw it.

The crushed ice in his ginger ale had started to melt.

THAT DAMN BELL

"I am ringing that damn bell today!" Jolene announced before I even made it through the doorway, her arms flailing like she'd been cooped up too long. I wasn't always assigned to Jolene, but fate put me there the day she rang the bell.

"Tara! I'm so glad I have you!" She reached to hug me. "I don't give a damn about six feet." She pulled me in—her blue eyes pierced through me, carrying all the color between her mask and the brim of her hat.

When cancer patients complete their treatment, they ring a bell to mark the moment—the closing of a chapter, the beginning of whatever comes next. At UPMC, the bell tolls for milestones, chemotherapy completion, personal victories—quiet triumphs that deserve to be heard. It rings loud and proud, met with cheers, tears, and sometimes...dancing.

We gathered around the bell, her family and friends clapping and ready for cheers. A phone blared Pharrell's feel-good anthem, *Happy*, and Jolene pulled me in, moving with ease as I stumbled alongside her. She danced up to the bell and slammed the rope into its side. The bell rang out, dissolving into cheers and music as Jolene flashed peace fingers into the camera.

She posted it on TikTok, sending the clip to staff. I cannot dance. I have no rhythm. But when colleagues approached me the next day, phones in hand, watching me stumble through my giraffe-like moves, I barely noticed. Instead, I saw our ear-to-ear smiles. Even through masks, we beamed.

WARRIOR TWO

The scent of incense cut through the thick air. My forehead rested on the mat as my arms stretched out overhead. Soft music played beneath the pitter-patter of bare feet on hardwood. My lower back surrendered into a gentle pull as I eased deeper into child's pose. I closed my eyes, and a bead of sweat trickled down my face.

A voice floated above the music. I glanced up from my mat, uncertain at first. The face didn't register, but the voice pierced through me—familiar in a way I couldn't place. *Sun Salutation A, then B. Warrior Three.* We moved. I searched. Who is she? She was with someone. Who?

By Warrior Two, my thighs burned and the floodgates opened.

Carol. Jack's wife.

It had been three years. The last time I saw her, it was the three of us. Carol never missed Jack's appointments. But now, she stood alone, holding onto Warrior Two.

When class ended, I approached her.

"Carol," I said with caution. I knew grief could make even a simple hello feel like intrusion.

"Yes," she said, squinting, the way people do when they're trying to pull a face from the fog.

"I was Jack's nurse at Hillman."

Her expression shifted, eyes lifted, widened. "Oh, Tara!"

She wrapped her arms around me, tight.

"I am so sorry, Carol," I whispered. "I was heartbroken to hear."

"Oh, he loved you. We loved you." Her tears welled, and something warm and broken passed between us. "I miss him every day," she said, voice thin with ache.

I nodded, letting silence carry the weight.

"How are the kids?" she asked, almost urgently, as if needing joy to break through. We talked about kindergarten, preschool, and Delaware—about life's new rhythms. She listened like always.

"I had to move too," she said. "The house held too much of him. But he still visits me."

I smiled. Of course he did.

"On his motorcycle," she added, grinning. "Tells me, 'Ride through it.' The grief, the discomfort, the whole damn mess."

"That was his line," I said, my lips curling into a knowing smile. We stood there in it for a moment. Then we stepped back into our own lives again.

47 STEPS

The June heat pressed in as we packed up the townhome. To my kids, this wasn't just a house—it was their first everything.

The stairs had memorized their tiny climbs. The windows had framed their wonder. They ran their hands along the walls like they were saying goodbye to something that had held them.

Boxes lined the floor. The boys bounced off each other like jelly beans. Trying to organize with them felt like mopping a flood with a sponge.

"Say goodbye, house. Thank you for serving us," I said, scanning the space—familiarity now stripped bare.

The boys paused, their big brown eyes flickering with curiosity. They knew we were moving, but I wasn't sure they grasped what that meant.

"Goodbye, house. I love you," Cooper shouted, sincerity tucked into every word.

Davey echoed him, then dove back into wrestling. Their laughter bounced off the bare walls.

I wanted to bolt—rush through the ache of goodbye. But something in me slowed.

"Let's go upstairs and say goodbye, boys," I said.

We climbed all 47 steps, their fingers trailing the walls, shouting goodbyes to every room like they were old friends. I paused in our empty bedroom, the room we brought our babies home to.

The walls here had seen it all: midnight feedings, Sunday snuggles, whispered fights, forgiveness.

And then it was time to go.

I smiled through a tear, knowing: Memories don't belong to places. They travel. They live in us. Dave stayed behind to finish the last of the move while I packed the boys and Dakota into the Jeep, their hair tousled, cheeks pink from the sun.

We hugged our friends tightly one last time.

"Until next time," we said, waving to the neighborhood.

Something bittersweet settled in as we drove away.

Home is with us.

I glanced in the rearview, caught between leaving and staying.

I left a job, too—six years of showing up, bearing witness, holding space. No goodbye party. No tears. No one seemed to notice when I left.

But the work—the work was always enough.

The patients still reached me. They always did.

And something in me knew it was time.

THE GRAY ZONE

There's a space in oncology that no one taught me about.

It isn't in the textbooks or the protocols or the laminated sheets taped to the medication room wall. But it was in my coworkers' eyes—that quiet, knowing look we traded when we all saw the same gap between can and should. It was the gray zone where medicine's momentum meets a patient's reality. We'd agree with a small nod, not because we had answers, but because there was nothing any of us could do beyond the job we were hired for.

As I grew as a nurse, I began noticing it more.

Not in one hospital or one infusion center, but everywhere I worked—different doctors, different systems, different zip codes, different coworkers' stories. It showed up in the quiet moments, the ones where the room felt too small for the weight of what we were doing.

She was in her seventies—sharp as a tack.

Knew every medication she took and why she took it. She lived alone, without a caregiver to help her navigate any of it.

She was one of many who lived in that gray zone between can and should.

Arthritis had stolen her mobility years before cancer arrived. An ambulance brought her to every treatment and took her home afterward.

Her regimen was aggressive—the kind built for younger bodies, stronger bodies, bodies with more margin. Curative intent, though.

But the day she was assigned to me, she was squeezed between two other patients who also needed my attention. One was nauseated and dehydrated. The other was anxious and new to treatment. All three deserved time, education, presence. But oncology doesn't always allow for that. The schedule was full. The chairs were full. The day was full.

To give her the education she needed—the kind that requires slowing down, sitting eye-level, asking real questions—felt impossible. I was already behind before I hung her first bag.

As I started her infusion, a question lodged itself in me—one that wouldn't let go.

She never complained.

She never questioned.

She trusted the plan because it was the plan.

But I watched her wince as she shifted in the bed and we placed her on the bedpan. I watched her hands tremble when we took the bedpan away—gowned and gloved, no one thinking about the chemotherapy vapors rising between us, just trying to get her clean and dignified.

And I felt it—that quiet moral ache.

We were pumping a cocktail of toxic drugs into a woman whose baseline quality of life was already fragile. We were following the protocol. We were doing what the system was built to do.

But I couldn't shake the feeling that we were missing something essential. Her voice. Her understanding. Her choice.

I didn't know if anyone had sat with her long enough to talk about goals of care. Not in the abstract, not in the "this is curative" sense, but in the real way. The way that asks:

What matters to you?

What does a good day look like?

What are you not willing to lose?

I didn't know if she knew she had a choice. And some patients don't even understand they have a choice, even when we tell them.

It wasn't a failure of anyone's care. It was the impossible tension between prolonging life and honoring the life being lived.

At the end of the day, when the call bells finally grew quiet and most of the nurses had already left, I stayed behind waiting for her ambulance. The unit felt softer then, dimmer, slower, almost like the building itself exhaled once the rush was over. With no one else tugging at my attention, we finally had space to talk.

She told me about her father and her aunt, and as she spoke, her eyes filled. Their relationships had been tender and steady—the kind that shapes a person long after the people are gone. It was clear she missed them both. Clear she yearned for company. Clear she carried her loneliness the same way she carried everything else—without complaint.

The awareness I'd been carrying for years stayed with me—into my drive home, into my shower, into the silent moments before sleep.

It wasn't guilt. It wasn't regret. It was awareness—the kind that changes you.

It was the moment I realized that oncology isn't just about medicine.

It's about meaning.

It's about alignment.

It's about making sure the treatment matches the life, not the other way around.

PART V

2022—LEWES, DELAWARE

TUNNELL CANCER CENTER

HALF A MILE AHEAD

The move to coastal Delaware was a leap of faith. We thought the coast would suit our lifestyle, and in some ways, it did. The beaches, the home, the community pool, the proximity to my parents—all draws. The coast offered beauty and ease, but we missed the mountains—the daily hikes, the scent of damp earth.

In Delaware, there was salt in the air, the crash of waves, and bright but unfamiliar mornings in our new home. We tried to savor the new experiences, even as nothing felt settled yet.

My new job took time to adjust to, as most do. It was in a small, overburdened infusion center—tucked between beach towns and retirement communities—that Delaware began to teach me how to see. The center was busy—stretched thin, always at capacity.

When I started, there were only two oncologists. Doctors treated every cancer type. The treating nurse sat among the patients.

Four chemotherapy chairs arranged in a rectangle, my computer on wheels floating in the center like a makeshift island.

At first, all I saw were the cracks: outdated chairs, a chaotic layout, a pharmacy where nurses primed the chemo lines. Dingy curtains that didn't quite close. An ancient computer system I already knew too well from UPMC. Some colleagues were friendly. Others barely offered a "good morning." The ambiance didn't hold a candle to the centers I'd known.

But the patients began to shift something in me.

"You're all so great," one man said.

"I just love this place," offered another.

"I hate having cancer, but I love coming here," said a woman, her smile radiant.

"You all make this easier."

Their words chipped away at my resistance—not because the chairs ever got replaced or the curtains fixed—but because their way of seeing began to change mine.

Then one sunny morning, Gus cracked me open.

He shuffled alongside me, his walker groaning with each uneven step. His gaze low, his hair thin and silver. His face held time.

"A while back," he said, "someone asked me to imagine walking through a forest."

He reached his chair and paused, eyes closed. I followed him.

"Now imagine a cliff at the end," he continued. "You can't see it yet, but it's there, about half a mile ahead."

I smiled—I liked a good cliff.

"That cliff is death," he said plainly.

He lowered himself into the chair. His voice was calm.

"Would you walk through that forest differently, knowing what's ahead?"

I nodded, throat tight. "Yes. I'd appreciate that walk a lot more."

Gus looked at me, his eyes fiery.

"Well, why the hell can't you all the time?"

Something in me opened, even if I didn't have language for it yet. I smiled. But I didn't answer.

His question stuck with me like a seed.

How do I walk like I know the cliff is there—and still notice the forest while I can?

That was the shift. The praise, the warmth—none of it was about walls or chairs or curtains.

It was about perspective.

They walked with awareness.

They knew the path was finite.

They noticed everything.

POCKETS IN TIME

I stood under the fireworks over Lewes Bay, and a thought rose that I couldn't shake.

There are these pockets in life—brief, golden stretches where everything aligns. A strong connection. A winning team. A group of moms raising babies as neighbors. A unit of coworkers who just get each other. The right people, the right energy, the right season.

And it is fleeting.

Maybe that's why it glows.

A year, maybe two. A stretch of golden weeks. A season, if you're lucky. Then someone moves. Someone graduates. Someone's life shifts. The moment dissolves.

But while it's happening, it's magic. You don't always know it at the time. Sometimes you only understand later how rare it was, how precise the timing had to be for it all to come together.

When I'm paying attention, I try to honor them. To name them. To hold them gently, like fireflies in a jar, knowing they were never meant to stay, only to glow for a while.

Maybe that's what life is. Not one long, continuous thread,

but a series of blips—perfect, fleeting alignments. And maybe the point isn't to hold on tighter but to notice when it's happening—to feel it, be in it, and let it go.

And perhaps, when they pass, they leave behind something more—a sense of what's worth chasing. A reminder that magic exists, and that we're allowed to want it again.

CHAIRLIFT

I asked my patient how she ended up owning a little clothing boutique on the coast.

She smiled, the sort of smile people give when they're glad you asked.

It was a simple question, the kind that opens a door without pushing it.

It reminded me of the way my father asks questions.

I can still picture us on chairlifts in the winter, strangers swinging beside him, the cold air carrying their voices.

By the time we reached the top, we'd know where they grew up, how they found their work, and what brought them to the mountain that day.

He never pried.

He just asked the kind of questions that made people feel like they mattered.

I didn't know I was learning anything at the time. I thought that was just how adults talked to each other. But now, years later, I hear his cadence in my own. The gentle curiosity. The way a single question can soften a room. The way people open up when they feel seen.

Sometimes I think my whole career has been one long chair-lift ride—a few minutes with someone suspended between where they've been and where they're going, and me beside them, asking just enough to understand who they are—and sometimes, who I am too.

STILL LOOKING

I confused Hank with another guy at first. I do that sometimes —giving a very generous wave and smile, greeting someone with the wrong name or someone else's backstory. More often than not, I'm met with a puzzled look, the kind that makes me immediately regret my enthusiasm. But Hank laughed hard when I mistook him for the number one runner in Delaware.

"Is that why you're so nice to me? You think I'm fast?" he enunciated fast with a deep chuckle.

"Speed never won me over, Hank, but humor always did." I met his grin with mine, already feeling the pull of his charm.

Hank spoke in a rhythm, his words unspooling effortlessly, like someone who told these stories a thousand times but still managed to keep them fresh.

"I moved to California at 23 to find myself." He glanced over one shoulder, then the other, as if scanning for the self he'd once misplaced. "And I'm still looking."

Hank was seventy-five.

I broke into a smile. "Aren't we all?"

He chuckled, lines etching deeper into his weathered face—the kind of laugh that had seen decades.

"So, how'd you end up in Delaware?" I asked, always curious about the paths that led people to new places. Maybe because I wasn't entirely sure how I'd ended up there myself.

"Oh, my wife wanted to be near family. But let me tell you, I was the only one moving from California to Delaware." His undertone made me smile. "I'd tell people we were moving to Delaware, and they'd say, 'where? Dela-where?'"

We laughed at the familiar joke for good reason.

"Delaware has three counties. California has fifty-eight!" He raised a brow, as if the statistic alone could explain everything. Hank continued, "We hated it. I traveled all the time for work—I got to leave." He laughed, like someone who'd long ago made peace with the choice. "There's just nothing here other than the wind and ocean," he said, effortlessly shifting gears. "So, what brought you here?"

Hank had a knack for balancing storytelling with curiosity, making sure the conversation wasn't one-sided.

"I'm still figuring that out, Hank," I answered, because the truth was still blurry around the edges.

Hank chuckled, shaking his head like he had already anticipated my response. "I picture you in the mountains. That's where people still move like they have legs that carry stories."

It was both a statement and a question. His eyes scanned my face, looking for confirmation.

I laughed, a little caught off guard by how close he'd landed. And I found myself wanting to linger—just to see what else he might notice.

THE CITY DOG

It was Cooper and Davey's fifth birthday when I volunteered to read to their class. The school gave parents the option: bring a book or be surprised. I liked surprises. But when the teacher handed me *A City Dog and a Country Frog*, the title caught me mid-motion—tugging loose a memory I hadn't touched in years.

It had been a long time since I'd really thought about Gail. After our last email exchange seven years earlier, the musical lamb she gave me made its way into Addison's newborn photo session, and I sent her a few pictures. She'd been thrilled to see the lamb beside my baby. She told me her scans showed no new cancer growth—stable disease. She was back at work but still receiving treatment.

I knew what "stable" meant. The cancer was at bay, but the cells remained, waiting and evolving. Still, at the time, she sounded hopeful. She wished me well on my motherhood journey and asked for more photos.

We moved twice after that. I'm not sure if the lamb came with us.

I never sent more pictures. Life got in the way; at least that's the excuse people use when we don't want to admit we forgot something that mattered.

I gathered myself and read the story to the class of four- and five-year-olds. It was about a city dog who befriends a frog in the countryside. They play through the seasons together until winter comes, and the frog doesn't return.

The kids made guesses about what happened. We talked about new friendships, about keeping old friends in our hearts while making new ones as the seasons change.

But the class consensus was firm: "The frog died." Children say the quiet part out loud, even when adults want to reshape the ending.

That night, at bedtime, Cooper started crying. He turned his back to me as I rubbed it gently beside him.

"What's wrong, Coop?" I asked.

Between soft sobs, he said, "I'm sad the frog died. Now the dog's all alone."

I nodded. "Yeah…it's hard to lose a friend."

I didn't mention the squirrel, the friend who came after the frog. Some friendships aren't meant to be replaced.

I rubbed his back, thinking about Gail.

The next day, I emailed her. I told her about the boys who entered our family five years earlier and about the strange irony of being handed that exact story she'd given me to read to their class. I apologized for not staying in touch and asked how she was, hoping for good news and a speedy reply.

I got neither.

But perhaps the story coming back to me was its own kind of reply.

SICK THIS MANY MONDAYS

When I was twenty-five, I compiled a list of the ten funniest people I knew. Friends and family jockeyed for position—clowning, campaigning, asking where they ranked.

Hank climbed that list fast.

"My son asked what I did all day at work," Hank said with a grin. "I told him, 'Son, I write emails. All day.'"

He asked, "I thought you worked in NYC?"

Hank dipped his head. "I said, 'Son, I do. And there—I write emails. All day.'"

We both smiled.

"I hated commuting into the city. Jersey to Manhattan—it wore me down, slow and brutal. I lost so much weight I thought I had cancer." He chuckled. "But it couldn't catch me back then."

It was rare for his diagnosis to surface in conversation. When it did, it slipped in sideways, tucked inside the punchline.

"Eventually, I got my commute down to Mondays only. Think about it—at least four holidays fall on a Monday. Christmas and New Year's can land on Mondays too."

He grinned.

"Then I'd say, okay…I can be sick this many Mondays."

I broke into a grin. Being near Hank was like watching a stand-up act.

"I need to get away from this drear." He kept going as I passed him his meds. "I told my wife—let's go to Bermuda. Get some sun."

"Great idea."

"She asked if I had a doctor's note." He paused, eyes narrowed in mock outrage.

"Who would you even give the note to?" I asked, teeing him up.

"Yeah," he said, gesturing like he was writing midair. "'Dear Mr. Pilot, please let this man fly on your airplane.'"

I laughed, loudly. Heads turned.

"Kids need doctor's notes." I wiped the tears in my eyes, a residual grin still playing on my face as I waited for more.

"I told my son," Hank continued, "and he said, 'Dad, I'll go with you.' So, we're going."

"That's great, Hank."

"Yeah...my scans are before we leave. If they're not good, I think I'll just stay there. I feel great. So, why not?"

My smile faltered. Hank's treatment plan was never curable; the goal was always to slow the growth of the cancer.

"I like that plan," I said, because what else was there to say.

We both looked past the room, toward something neither of us could name.

DETOX

The wind off the water bit at my skin. Dakota trotted ahead, tail high, nose to the ground. I was two days into a detox—no food, no intense exercise, no noise. Just walks by the water and whatever surfaced when I stopped numbing. It started with two days of shakes, then five days of easing food back in. My stomach growled, loud and insistent, protesting the silence too.

Siena got me into quarterly detoxes. Clear out the toxins. Help prevent the cancerous cells from replicating. I liked the ritual of it. There was something about the discipline—stripping away, resisting the urge to fill my body the moment hunger struck—that built me up. It felt like practice. Not just for health, but for presence and gratitude.

My phone buzzed. Shannon.

She lived in Peru, her second year. I always admired how easily she moved, how lightly she carried place—how home was never trapped between the same walls or people.

Her voice crackled through the patchy signal. "It's not very comfortable here," she said, and I nodded as my stomach growled. "The homes are big enough for sleep and shelter. And small enough that people get outside."

I pictured her on a dusty street, laundry flapping, voices rising and falling like music. "It's a different way of living," she added. "More of a needs-based life. It's simpler. Not easy, but I actually think I like it better."

Her words felt like part of the detox. In Peru, simplicity wasn't a trend—it was a way of life. No curated pantries, no overflowing carts. Just enough. In the United States, we call it consumption. We say "need" when we mean "want." We fill space to avoid feeling empty.

I was trying to do the opposite. Strip back. Sit with the ache. Let hunger teach me something.

We didn't talk long. Shannon was already halfway to the next thing—a bike tour, a pulse of motion I couldn't match.

After we hung up, I kept walking. I thought about the small homes filled with Peruvian food and love. In Delaware, the neighborhood felt still, like everyone was careful not to ripple the surface.

The wind picked up. Dakota chased a sandpiper into the surf.

The horizon blurred where the ocean met the sky—soft, transient, always becoming something else.

I kept walking.

Walks, water, walks by the water. Not to escape the hunger but to learn to carry discomfort.

ONE AND DONE

Leni sat stone-faced, staring past the rows of chairs into the open space of the cancer center. Her eyes held an emotion that words couldn't capture. At Tunnell Cancer Center, nurses ran pre-infusion checks. I double-checked the essentials.

"How are you feeling today?" The question felt hollow the moment it left my mouth.

"Edgy and anxious. You?" she shot back, her voice clipped.

My lips tightened. A volunteer offered her a snack, but she declined. Silence stretched, thick with tension.

"Any nausea or fatigue?" I asked, defaulting to protocol.

Her expression stayed fixed. "I keep thinking about all the side effects and whether I even want these drugs."

I hesitated.

"This is my first treatment," she snapped.

I froze. I hadn't known. And suddenly, everything felt heavier.

Heat crawled up my neck. I hadn't reviewed her chart thoroughly enough. That kind of oversight chips away at trust. When care feels generic, so do we.

"I really feel like leaving," she said.

I did too.

"I'm sorry, Leni. Let me take a minute to review your chart more thoroughly."

She nodded, but I could feel her faith in the system slipping.

Six months earlier, Leni had felt a lump. Her doctor ordered the wrong kind of mammogram—a screening instead of a diagnostic—so she was sent home and told to start over. The delay cost her time she didn't have. By the time she was diagnosed, the cancer had already spread to her lymph nodes. Stage III. Urgent.

"I don't want any of that information. I know my options—treatment or die." She looked straight at me. "But I didn't want to come today." There was something lighter in her voice now. Not joy, but wry honesty.

"I'm sure this is all a lot." My words felt rehearsed. "Do you want to discuss your hesitation with our nurse practitioner?"

Leni's gaze narrowed. "Everyone just passes the buck around here."

She paused. My shoulders tightened.

"I don't want another doctor. I want to talk to you."

I shifted in my stool, aware of the delicacy of the moment. It happened sometimes. Patients consult the doctor, sign the consent, and still need a moment to catch up to the decision.

"This decision is yours. But…I can give you the information."

I explained the drugs and their side effects. The rhythm of labs, visits, and infusions.

Her treatment plan was considered curative, though the road would feel long—and might involve long-term medications and monitoring.

Her eyes softened.

"If you were me, what would you do?"

After more than a decade in oncology, the question still startled me. I'd thought about it before. But never long enough to let it settle.

I exhaled. "The drugs and the side effects sound scary," I said. "But I'd want to take that stake toward survival."

It wasn't advice. It was a glimpse into my own lens. Perspective is like slipping on someone else's prescription glasses. I might make something out—but it's a distorted lens, shaped by the people I love, the fears I carry, and the things I stand to lose.

She said she pictured me going home to my kids and the chaos of our big dog—something unexpectedly accurate.

I smiled—for the first time all conversation. "You're good," I said—and meant it.

"I'm right?"

Her shoulders relaxed. She sensed something true. I let it land.

"My will to live is different. My husband never wanted children. I've been on birth control since I was a teenager. I blame that for my cancer." Her words held grief over the nonchoices that brought her here.

She looked past me, past the rows of chairs, into something deeper.

"I never thought about my health until now," she said quietly. "You don't realize what you have until it's threatened."

I nodded, knowing all too well the health I took for granted —not intentionally. Just in the way that wellness lets you look away.

"My passion is mountain biking," she said. "We do it all the time—we even travel for it." She paused, her jaw tight. "What if I'm too tired to do the things I love?"

Treatment can take more than illness. Leni wasn't ready to lose herself. And she was still young enough to fight for more than just time.

"That's a real fear," I said gently. "And it matters. Treatment might ask a lot, but you can protect the parts of you that make you feel like yourself."

Something shifted. Her shoulders eased.

"You have a calming demeanor," she said. "I feel less anxious." She studied me, still weighing her options. "I may be one and done," she finally said. "But let's do this today."

I nodded, watching Leni sit with her decision.

We tried to smile, but it didn't hold.

WILD AND SUN-BLEACHED

Their blond hair was wild and sun-bleached from summer on the coast, ticking up in every direction—the kind of feral chaos only five-year-olds can pull off. Their backpacks bounced as they walked toward the school doors, small bodies moving with that mix of confidence and hesitation that comes with doing something big for the first time.

I stood there watching them go, feeling the moment stretch.

And then it hit me: Maya was a kindergarten teacher.

She would have been the kind of teacher who saw them the way she once saw me—fully, without rushing, without missing the small magic.

I felt the ache and the gratitude rise together, the way they always did with her. For a moment, it was as if she were beside me again, reminding me to stay awake to the world.

Cooper turned back and blew me a kiss, and I reached for it.

A BOOK THAT GREW IN SAND

The place that dulled me gave shape to the thing I was meant to write. Maybe it was the thinning of connection. The boys off to kindergarten, the days stretching open. The quiet, finally.

The house settled into a new rhythm. Motherhood stopped being the whole day and became just parts of it.

We moved to Delaware to be closer to my parents and to keep things afloat with young children and a new zip code. The misalignment showed up slowly—a sense of being slightly off-axis.

Not to write a book.

But over the years, I had been writing down the stories—scribbled in notebooks, stored in digital files, tucked into memory for safekeeping. For years, they sat. And the silence of Lewes stirred them to life. It felt fluid against the flatness of the place. The conversations, the casual, neighborly ones—pleasant enough but thin.

First in pieces. Maya. Maureen. Siena. The city dog and the country frog.

Then Tiny. Benny. Hank. The patients who lingered in my

mind long after I clocked out. The ones who rearranged me. I wanted to hold their stories, even if I wasn't sure what for.

Eventually, I read one aloud to the staff. Someone said, "You should publish that." Someone else nodded and said, "That's exactly how I felt." They leaned closer. They asked for more.

And the words kept coming. Sometimes between infusions. Sometimes in the back row of staff meetings. Sometimes by the ocean, scribbled into the spine of a damp notebook while the kids chased waves and Dakota dozed in the sand.

Delaware became home in every way that mattered.

Not because it dazzled, but because it held still long enough for me to listen. It became the place where this book began to stretch its spine.

It started in fragments.

It started in salt.

It started.

LIKE A TAPESTRY

Doctors told Susan she had three to six months to live. The diagnosis came just weeks after she and her husband retired to the beach.

Susan sat before me, calm and serene. Fine lines framed her eyes and mouth. A book rested in her lap. She looked younger than the 68 listed on her chart.

"They were like stair steps—born back-to-back," she said, telling me about her four adult children. She chuckled, then paused as a tear slipped into the folds of her sweatshirt.

"I'm sorry," she said. "I can talk about anything but my children without crying."

"Oh, I understand," I said. "That's hard." Life can turn fast. Something in me tightened—the way it does when motherhood brushes up against loss.

"I think this will be my last treatment. I just wanted to make it through the holidays," she said. "I want my children to enjoy them—without remembering them as the season I died."

It was three weeks before Christmas. Even in her dying, she was trying to make it easier for them to live.

"I don't want chemo to be the thing that takes me down. I've lived a good, full life."

The tears returned. I reached for tissues.

"Why did you choose oncology?" she asked after a pause, her eyes curious. "This must be so hard—treating all these weepy people like me."

We laughed, breaking the heavy.

"It can be," I said. "But I like hearing people's stories."

She chuckled. "That's why my daughter chose the ER."

I grinned. "Yeah. The opposite of this."

I let the pause breathe.

"Well, it must be hard," she said softly. "Thank you for doing what you do. You get to know my story…and then, well—I won't be here for us to continue getting to know each other."

"It can be," I admitted. "But most of my patients are… refreshing to be around. There's a raw sense of being alive."

Her expression shifted, and I felt myself stop.

"I don't mean to sound like your loss is my gain," I said gently.

"I didn't feel that," she replied. Her eyes softened, almost sad.

"I don't know if you ever soften things," I said, "but this conversation—it's open, honest. That's why I chose oncology. These moments carry into the way I live."

She smiled. Then, after a beat: "Like a tapestry."

I tilted my head.

"I sew," Susan smiled. "And conversations…they ebb and flow like threads."

I nodded, drawn to the metaphor instantly.

"They weave through the fabric," she added. She was right. Conversations connect us, stitching things together in ways we don't notice at the time.

"Yes," I said. "I try to carry these conversations into the rest of my life."

"They change the pattern," she said softly.
And we let the moment settle.

A SPOT ON THE LIST

"It was just breathtaking," Hank began as he settled into my section, already diving into storytelling. He always carried the same book on the Battle of Normandy. It became a running joke between us. He claimed the hefty book was a prop to avoid conversations with people—his bookmark always in the same spot.

"You can feel the history there and see the remnants of war. It was the trip of a lifetime." As Hank spoke, tears gathered in his eyes. I grew confused. He'd been excited to talk about this trip a moment ago. His voice became a tremor. "I'm sorry—the pollen," he chuckled, covering tears he pretended weren't there. I extended a box of tissues.

"I'm sorry, Hank. Are you okay?"

"Yeah, the trip was a couple of years ago; I don't know exactly when. You know I'm terrible with timetables." I smiled. I knew that about Hank. I knew a lot about Hank from the small window we shared.

"My brother-in-law planned it; he and I were close. He was pretty sick, but that trip was his last good leg. He didn't make it much longer after that. He had cancer too." Hank's eyes welled. "I'm sorry," he said, a flush rising. "This pollen *is* bad today."

I chuckled. "Oh...please don't apologize, Hank. It's okay to cry." I fumbled, reaching for the tissue box.

My words hung in the thick air. The quiet was too loud. "My sons say their tears aren't real sometimes too." I smirked, hoping to lighten the moment.

Hank chuckled. "You mean your six-year-olds?"

I could only laugh. His voice regained its confidence. "Maybe because our squished crying faces are pretty ugly. I mean, really, it's hardly flattering—that contoured face, running slimy fluid everywhere."

Our laughter collided with the tears. I inhaled, breath hitching.

"So, where am I on your list?" Hank beamed.

"Oh, Hank, you're definitely number one today."

Hank's smile widened.

RIPRAP

We got a letter from the HOA about the kids being by the pond. The letter used the word 'riprap.'

I had to Google it. It's the rocky edge around a pond. It preserves the fragile ecosystem of the man-made pond. My children's proximity to it was a violation.

"They were seen throwing large pieces of ice onto the pond." The pond was frozen. They threw ice onto ice. In winter.

The HOA was worried about my kids' safety—which I sort of understood—and about protecting the pond, which felt like Mother Nature's territory.

I screenshotted the letter and sent it to Meg.

She replied, "Fragile ecosystem? It's a retention pond, not the Galápagos."

I laughed.

"Did they mean riffraff?"

I thought that too.

"Who are these people? Don't they have jobs?"

I chuckled. It was easier to laugh.

"The HOA leader knocked on our door on a Monday morning."

There was a pause. Then Meg, in her signature tone: "Someone leads?"

I laughed again.

"I live in a place that has a riprap rule."

"Yeah. That's no way to live."

Another flicker of misalignment.

MORE DEATH VISITS

Ray bled positive energy. He and his wife sat before me, all smiles. The nurse giving me report believed he'd gotten bad news, that he was out of treatment options. But with their smiles still painted across their faces, she wasn't entirely sure. And neither was I.

"Ray, nice to meet you. I'm Tara."

"Oh, we've met before, Tara. Come on. I'm a dying man. Act like you remember my handsomeness."

I smiled, uneasy. "I remembered you."

"People are surprised when I tell them I'm dying," he said, lips straightening. "But I've lived a good life."

"That's great you feel that way," I said, my voice unsteady, unsure if it was the right thing to say.

His phone binged. He craned his neck to check it.

"More death visits," he said, deadpan.

"People want to see you."

"Yup. They need closure on our time together." He smiled. "Everyone's dropping everything to come say goodbye. Then they take one look at me and say, 'You're not dying.'"

Ray was with me for two units of red blood cells—his last.

He'd asked for them not to prolong anything, but to stay steady long enough for one final meal with friends and family. He knew sustaining life wasn't realistic anymore.

Myeloma patients often look well, even vibrant, while needing frequent transfusions just to stay afloat. The cancer crowds out the bone marrow—the body's cell factory. When transfusions become daily and can no longer hold the line, patients begin to feel it—the slow slip in quality of life.

Some resist that truth. Others, like Ray, reach an acceptance.

"This myeloma made me a better man," he said, looking up. "I'm humbler. A lawyer by trade, I was arrogant. It was hard for me not to be in control. My firm, my staff, everything I oversaw —it was all about control." He paused, then smiled. "I was a damn good lawyer," he said. "But this cancer...it wasn't like a big tumor they could cut out of me. Everything I thought I had power over disappeared the moment my health was on the line."

Silence settled between us. I wished for something wise to say, but nothing came. My head bobbed like a buoy.

"I guess it's hard to accept what we can't control," I said, unsure if it helped.

Ray nodded. "And harder to change what we can."

"And wisdom to know the difference," his wife finished, like it was something they'd said before.

We'd spoken the Serenity Prayer without meaning to.

"Why does it take something like this?" I still couldn't use the word 'dying,' as if it were a secret we were all pretending not to know.

Ray's wife mirrored my head bobbing, her smile unshaken.

"Because we think we have all the time in the world to see each other."

"I've lived a great life, though. I have no regrets," Ray repeated.

And somehow, in one shift, he got under my skin.

Just by being himself, all the way through. His jokes—sometimes relentless—still softened the edges. His smile didn't waver, even as his body did. He wasn't fighting death. He was making room for it.

I didn't have the right words when we hugged goodbye. Just a quiet nod, and the weight of what we both knew.

His wife's eyes filled when she hugged me too, the emotion finally breaking through.

HERON POINT

Cape Henlopen became our spot. A golden-hour ritual built not out of tradition but necessity—the day's heat softened, the kids were looser, the beach nearly empty.

We always set up near the jetty at the north end, where the skimboarders danced across the surf like water bugs. We stood in the sand watching them cut and spin. That stretch of beach felt different—rugged and restless. The dunes behind us stood tall and curved, like they were leaning into the water. You could almost hear them whispering, "Climb me." Signs said otherwise, of course. Delaware loved its signage. NO dogs off leash. Absolutely NO fishing in the pond. NO climbing on the dunes. But temptation was part of our landscape.

Dave would wander the shoreline with Dakota off-leash, chasing the sandpipers. The boys sprinted feral loops around us. Addison and I had a game we'd played since she could walk: run into the ocean, then back out before a wave could catch us. The boys joined in. Their shriek-laughter, the soaked shorts, the feeling of almost outrunning something larger than us. It never got old. And we lost, sometimes. And somehow, that's when we felt most alive.

Later, as the sun dipped lower, Cooper and Davey began dragging their hands and heels across the smooth, damp sand. They didn't speak, just moved, mirroring each other like twin calligraphy. Addison and I watched as they worked their way toward the center of the shape, meticulous and absorbed. I climbed the rocks for a better view.

From above, it was a perfect monkey head. One side drawn with hands and heels, the other with heels and hands—meeting right in the middle.

No discussion necessary. Just instinct and symmetry.

We weren't rooted there. Not really. Delaware didn't quite hold that for me. But in moments like this, it didn't matter. We weren't waiting for it to feel like home. We were just together—outrunning waves, sketching animals in the sand, chasing sandpipers.

Content anyway.

OLIE

Dannie was on cycle six of seven in her treatment for ovarian cancer. At 75, she wore a flashy yellow top hat with a fake flower on the rim—an eclectic touch that matched her personality.

I'd been her nurse many times, just not that day. Her stories were long and winding, especially on days when my own energy was thin.

Her nurse was hooking up the infusion when I stepped over to check on the patient beside her. I overheard her say, "This drug can cause allergic reactions."

Dannie looked up from her handbag, pulling out a rosary. "Like what would I feel?"

"Shortness of breath, lower back pain. Some patients just say, 'I feel funny.' Let me know if you feel anything different at any point."

She nodded, her fingers tightening around the rosary.

I moved to the next chair. Olie—the black lab therapy dog—stood in my path, his volunteer handler chatting nearby. I gave him a quick rub and slipped past.

I was mid-assessment when Olie suddenly bolted. I'd never seen him move like that.

I turned—Dannie's face was bright red.

Her nurse ran to her pump and called for help. I placed an oxygen mask around her face. Olie stayed close. Through Dannie's fear, a faint smile surfaced.

He held his stance. Steady. As if this was the job he was called to do.

The nurse practitioner arrived, and we worked around Olie's broad frame. Slowly, the color returned to Dannie's face.

She blinked, then turned toward the volunteer. "Did you just say Olie?"

"Yes, Olie," he said, gently tugging the leash.

Dannie hesitated, her voice shaky. "That was my father's name."

I felt goosebumps rise along my arms.

Olie's owner paused, then spelled it out. "O-L-I-E. Not many people spell it like that."

Dannie inhaled sharply. "That's how my father spelled his name." Tears brimmed in her eyes.

She smiled, her face returning to its original color. She cupped Olie's face, searching for his eyes. "He always told me he would visit me when I needed him."

I blinked, not surprised by the sting—just grateful I hadn't grown numb to it yet.

I'd come to expect the unexpected in oncology—reactions, losses, miracles.

But this felt like something else.

NO CELL PHONES IN HEAVEN

We still had plenty of day left when the kids piled on me. Cooper wedged a book into my hand. Davey dove in from the other side. Addison clawed for a bit of mommy real estate. Even Dakota circled at my feet, eager to absorb the excitement and claim a piece of the lovefest. They piled on, and I let the moment hold me.

I wished I could bottle it, seal it tight, and borrow from it on harder days. Short of that, I wanted our time together to mean something. I opened the book, barely finishing the first sentence before elbows flew. I fought for breath under the crush of affection.

"Let's go outside," I said—my go-to fix for everything.

Within minutes, we were airborne, feet hitting the trampoline, laughter rising into the afternoon. Endorphins soared. Cortisol plummeted.

Our medicine is outdoor time and boredom—the things that bring us back to each other.

I see it at work—at the bedside, the chairside—the love that shows up, and the love that doesn't. The love we get and the love we give.

And in the end, who doesn't want a full heart and a lap full of company?

That evening, we went out to dinner—a rare occasion for my rowdy bunch—and Addison and I walked to the bathroom together.

As I waited for her, I scrolled my phone for no good reason.

"Mommy, are you still there?" her small voice called through the stalls.

I was.

"Yup, right here."

I looked up and caught my reflection in the mirrors above the sink—surprised by the grown-up staring back at me. The child long faded. Aging's gradual transformation had snuck in.

Had I savored enough?

Music in the background slipped through my fog.

Bare Necessities played over the restaurant sound system.

The song was almost over.

"Mommy." Addison was smiling up at me.

"Why are you crying?"

I glanced at my reflection, tears blending with mascara.

I hummed the familiar, catchy tune—the one about letting go of the extra and holding onto what's essential—and smiled at Addison as she twirled to the beat.

"Happy tears, hon. A good friend used to play this for me on her guitar."

Addison's big blue eyes filled with curiosity.

"What's her name?"

"Maya."

"Where is she?"

"Oh…she's in Heaven now, honey. Telling me to slow down."

Addison smirked, eyeing the phone in my hand.

"I tell you that, too, Mom," she said.

"You do."

She slipped her small fingers around mine, tugging my hand away from the screen as she skipped ahead.

"There are no cell phones in Heaven," she added.

And even after a decade of watching the threat of death change the way people live, I still needed reminders of what it looks like to be alive.

THE HARD ONE

In oncology, most patients humble me. They arrive cracked open—by diagnosis, by fear, by love—and they let me in.

But every nurse eventually meets the one who doesn't—the one who makes you question not your clinical skills, but your emotional endurance.

Johnathon was sitting upright, waving me over for the third time, eyes fixed on me like I'd kept him waiting—even though we'd just been together minutes earlier.

"Where are my meds?" he said, pointing to the empty IV pole like it would help expedite the process.

"Pharmacy's mixing them," I said, trying not to let my irritation show. "They'll send them as soon as they're ready." He knew the process, he just didn't like it.

His face tightened. "So can't you call them and tell them to hurry up? Why wasn't it done sooner?"

I felt the familiar tug—the urge to explain, to soften, to make it easier. But I had three other patients who needed drugs hung, pumps checked, symptoms assessed—patients who weren't taking their frustration out on me. I didn't have time to cushion something I couldn't change.

"You can talk to my manager if you'd like," I said, something I almost never do. He kept arguing, but I stepped out before the guilt could catch up to me.

My manager stepped in as I moved to the patient beside him. He didn't back off right away; it took time for the edge in his voice to fade.

Johnathon didn't want to connect. He wanted to control. His questions weren't curious; they were combative. He scrutinized every detail, dismissive of the care around him, indifferent to the dozen other patients we were tending.

After my shift with him, I left brittle.

I sat in my car longer than usual, hands still tight on the steering wheel. It wasn't his anger that got to me—it was the way it made me doubt myself, the way it scraped at the part of me that wants to be steady for everyone. I felt wrung out, like I'd poured from a cup that was already empty. And for a moment, I wondered if I was cut out for this kind of day.

But I finally realized boundaries are not the opposite of care—they are care.

MACHU PICCHU

It was summer again when I found myself thinking about Leni.

A year had passed since her first treatment—the last time I saw her. We never crossed paths again, but her story stayed with me. I still hoped her journey was unfolding somewhere. Maybe she'd chosen a different cancer center. Or maybe she'd chosen an entirely different path. Wherever she is, Leni taught me something I hadn't expected: clarity doesn't always come from fighting.

We're so often told, "Don't give up." "Give it your all." But what if "giving it your all" isn't a relentless struggle? What if it's riding life out on the backside of Machu Picchu—letting the journey dictate the fight rather than the other way around?

There's something healing in that possibility, too.

BOOKMARKS

It was nothing like our fresh-air hikes, but Siena and I scheduled check-in calls every few months. Our conversations were always like hitting the reset button, picking up where the last chapter left off. Seamless.

"So, how is life in Delaware?" Siena asked, her voice warm with that special sincerity only she could offer.

"Oh, you know. It still doesn't feel like home," I admitted. "But the kids are settled. Summer's beautiful here."

It had been two years. The settling-in period was long over. But some places never quite settle into you.

"I mean, our house is great," I added. "But everything else still feels slightly off. And the HOA's not exactly kid-friendly."

Siena didn't rush to fix it. She never did. She offered a few gentle thoughts—the kind that came from remembering something hard, but not being afraid of it anymore.

"Once you look past the discomfort," she said, "there's usually something to take from it."

We let that sit.

Sometimes there's no big revelation—just a friend who

reminds you that even when you don't know why you're somewhere, or how long you'll stay, you're still becoming something in the process.

THE MAN IN THE DRIVEWAY

Dave stood in the driveway, orange flip-flops on, swinging his golf club. For a moment, I saw the man I met before the blur of babies and bedtimes.

It was rarely just Dave and me anymore—we were mostly a family of five, all together.

I wondered if I was as lost to motherhood as we were to our marriage—each child reshaping me, reshaping us.

But we tried. We found each other on dinner dates, ski trips, rare nights alone. I was learning how to be present in a life that had arrived faster than I expected.

In three years, I met, married, and brought three children into the world with Dave. It could have been too much for two people still getting to know each other.

But so far, it's worked.

I've seen things fall apart in an instant. But I've also seen them come together just as fast.

That's the part we forget.

That's the part I want to remember.

WHERE BLUEBIRDS FLY

"We have a bell ringer!" a nurse called out. I swiveled around, eager to witness one of my favorite ceremonies.

Rita stood before the bell, all smiles. A sage bonnet covered her bare head. Her face softened into something bright.

I knew her backstory—three generations of breast cancer before her. A grandmother who'd had a radical mastectomy, a mother who died at 45, a great-grandmother lost young to what was almost certainly cancer.

Her friend raised the camera. "Ready!"

With trembling hands, Rita grasped the bell's roped handle. The metal vibrated under her touch. Empathy and hope surfaced—the battles fought, the nausea, the fatigue, the uncertainty. She looked free now—I hoped—in the only way you can be after all that.

The crowd erupted in applause. Even patients who might never ring the bell themselves lit up with shared smiles and tears.

"I'm going to sing everyone a little song," Rita announced.

The room stilled.

She began softly, her voice stealing the air. I didn't recognize the opening lines, but the melody carried a kind of ache—the kind that makes people lift their heads, lower their phones, close their eyes. A few nurses beside me smiled, humming along, already knowing where the song was headed.

Her voice grew stronger, filling the space. Patients at the edges of the room leaned in. I felt the pull of it too—the way a familiar tune can feel like a hand on your back.

Then she reached the part everyone knew.

A ripple went through the room—recognition, nostalgia, longing—and I felt tears gather before I could stop them. The melody tugged me backward—to nights when I held a baby in each arm, turning the dial on the lamb-shaped sound machine, singing softly into the dark. Six years ago, but it felt like another lifetime.

Rita kept singing, her voice rising and falling with a kind of courage that made my throat tighten. The room became a chorus—nurses, patients, caregivers—all of us blending into something imperfect and beautiful. No one cared about pitch. We cared about hope.

When she reached the part about bluebirds flying—the ache to rise above and beyond the storm—she lingered there, her voice catching at the edges. I looked around. Eyes brimmed everywhere.

For a moment, we were all dreaming of that place beyond pain, beyond fear, beyond the limits of our bodies. I wished for every patient to fly away from the pain, the disease. It felt impossible.

And then I realized we call that place Heaven.

THE HERMIT CRABS

It was a Monday in early fall. I was accessing her port when she asked, "So what'd you and the kids do this weekend?"

Elena asked about my kids with real curiosity—the kind that remembers names and quirks.

"We went to the beach," I said. "The kids brought their hermit crabs." She raised an eyebrow and chuckled. "You brought hermit crabs to the beach? Oh, I love that."

"Well...it was slightly traumatizing." My face dropped. She lifted her eyebrow again. "They wanted to let them explore the sand," I said. "We took them to the jetty. The crabs were climbers—one was halfway up a rock face, clinging to the side." I shaped the moment with my hands—one a rock, the other a crab. "And then, without warning, a wave slammed into us. The tide turned faster than I could react."

She laughed. "Oh no, I'm so sorry I'm smiling."

"My daughter grabbed hers. My sons' crabs vanished. I ran up and down the jetty, peering between rocks, calling for crabs. The kids were crying. It was so sad. I felt terrible."

Elena half-smiled. "No, no, I think they'll be all right. Crabs are meant for the sea, right?"

"You think?" I asked, half wanting to believe it. "We went back that evening at low tide, hoping to find them. A long shot, but we had to try."

She smirked. "Yeah, I think they're where they belong now."

"Yeah?"

She nodded. "I do. I'll look it up while I'm here," she said, already lifting her phone. I could've done the same, but I didn't have the heart to.

We talked a little more—about the crabs, about how kids hold onto hope longer than adults do, about her golf game.

When I deaccessed her port, I asked, "So? What'd you find out about those hermit crabs?"

She smiled. "Oh yeah…they'll be fine. They're where they belong." She gave a small wave, eyes on her things.

A few days passed. I kept thinking about those crabs and how quickly things can vanish. The boys brought them up now and then, their voices soft, their eyes wet. They kept asking if they were okay. I kept hoping Elena was right.

Eventually, I looked it up. Hermit crabs don't swim. They drown.

Elena had lied to me.

When I saw her weeks later, she smiled and said, "I thought it was better that way."

I didn't argue. Because maybe it was. Maybe the truth wouldn't have helped my children sleep. Maybe it wouldn't have helped me either.

Elena knew what I needed in that moment—what we all need sometimes. Not facts. Not fixes. Just a little softness. And a little hope.

THE BIKE

I turned the resistance knob and climbed. The stories came with me.

The pedals turned. My breath caught. Somewhere between the climb and the cooldown, the stories ignited and the book started talking back—like wildfire.

Scenes surfaced mid-sweat. Dialogue spilled out—words I couldn't reach when I was sitting still.

It wasn't silence that stirred creativity. It was motion that shook loose the stories piling inside, waiting for space to surface and take shape.

I used to think creativity came from slowing down. Maybe it also comes from rhythm. In this new quiet, I noticed everything. The way Dakota curled into the sun patch by the door. The way the light hit the monkey bars at 9:17 a.m. The way my body still held stories. My breath carried them. In the rhythm of movement, they finally found their way to the page.

I turned the resistance knob and climbed.

THE EDITOR

Robin was deep in conversation with Hank when I walked back in. She laughed hard, her voice cutting through the air and turning heads in my section. Hank was mid-performance, hands gesturing wildly.

"...then I'd say, okay—I can be sick this many Mondays."

I half-smiled at Hank's repeated story. It was a good one—maybe a little stretched—but his delivery always won the crowd.

I logged back into my computer as Robin looped me in.

"We were just talking about—wait, what are you writing? A book?"

I turned, confused, and found Robin peering over my shoulder. My screen displayed my writing. Despite the interruptions, I sometimes wrote at work. I considered lying, keeping the book close to my chest. *What if it never manifests once I say it out loud?*

"I am," I said, fighting the instinct to hide behind my masks.

"No way." Hank's excitement was palpable. "Fiction? Non-fiction?"

"Non-fiction."

"Is it about this?" Robin pointed toward the cancer center. She'd been an oncology nurse for over a decade; she knew. "This place is in need of some story-telling."

"I thought so too." Confidence stirred within our little trio.

Robin was intense, with a jarring boldness—a bluntness I loved, maybe because I carried so little of it myself.

"That's great," Hank said, smiling. I waited for him to make a joke of it. But he didn't.

"I'll say I knew you back when," Robin laughed, but my confidence thinned under the spotlight.

"It's really just something I enjoy doing," I hedged. "I'm not sure it'll amount to anything."

"Well, not with that attitude," Robin shot back, never one to let uncertainty go unchecked.

"How do you even publish a book?" Hank asked.

"I don't even know, Hank. That's how far I am from that." I laughed, but he held a curious expression.

"Who's looking at it for you? I was an English major," he said, eyebrows lifted in a confident smile.

"How convenient," Robin smirked, her arms swaying between us, creating an almost physical energy.

I chuckled, feeling my storytelling gain purpose.

Hank shifted in his chair. "I'm all yours." Then, with an easy chuckle—half serious, half joking—he added, "But you know my timeline is one big question mark."

"Thanks, Hank," I said, my thoughts spinning. I felt awkward accepting his offer, but I loved the idea. I shifted my weight, clasping my hands, nervous at the proposition.

"So...how about this weather?" I offered, grasping for neutral ground.

The three of us laughed small talk away.

"You're better than that," Robin smirked.

That night, I went home loving the idea of sending Hank my first chapter. Everyone needs an editor.

I placed the opening chapters in a folder.

And the folder felt so light, despite the heaviness it held.

COASTAL BISTRO

We gathered in the back room of a coastal bistro, tucked behind a brick wall that had probably heard a lot over the years. The air smelled like shellfish and wine. Nurses, out of scrubs and out of the rhythm of alarms, charting, and grief. It was rare to see us like this. Not rushing. Not solving. Just eating warm food and letting laughter in.

Elena had passed a few weeks earlier. Her partner dropped off gift bags for two other nurses and me. Management combined the gift cards for a staff outing.

Candlelight flickered against the glassware as I lifted my glass.

"Let's remember why we're here."

I stood before I could talk myself out of it. I hated public speaking. But it was my moment to give voice to the words I'd been writing for years.

"I want to pay tribute to Elena—the reason we're all here tonight," I said, my voice steadier than I felt.

I told them about the stories she shared: her childhood in Boston, her early retirement, her golf games, her travels. She asked about me, too—my family, my weekends, my trips. Our conversations were real. No pretending. No guard. There were laughs. There were tears.

On our last encounter, she asked, "How do you do this? Isn't this hard?"

"The loss never gets any easier," I answered.

"Well then why do you come back?" she asked, her eyes holding something like gratitude.

"Because I get to know people like you."

Elena smiled.

"I sometimes wonder if I made any difference to the patients who made a difference to me," I said to the crowd of coworkers, feeling confident in my closing. "But that's all I can really know for sure—their light, it changed me."

The room applauded. People wiped their eyes. Nurses came up to me, one after another.

"Write the book," Robin said. "You had me in tears."

"You should public speak," another said, pulling me into a hug.

I smiled. "Thank you. Thank you, guys."

They didn't just applaud the story. They handed me the strength to keep telling it.

And maybe that was Elena's final gift—the nudge to speak aloud what I'd only ever written down.

I'LL BE IN TOUCH

I approached the nurses' station just as Hank strolled into the infusion center. He wore the same worn-out yellow ball cap he always did, gripping the hefty Normandy book I never saw him without. He looked like he was about to make me laugh all afternoon.

"I'll take Hank today," I told the charge nurse.

It was the first time I claimed a patient. The words felt strange, but Hank was already grinning.

"Did you just pick me?" His smile stretched wide as he pointed to his chest.

"I sure did, Hank. I'm due for some laughs."

"Oh, the pressure's on—what's my status on your funny list anyway?" he asked, still smiling.

"Oh, you're up there, Hank—number three. Just something to keep you working for," I said with a smirk.

Hank's shoulders lifted with pride as he placed his book on his lap.

"Same spot as last week," he said, pointing to his bookmark. We chuckled.

"You need a new book."

It was my perfect segue to ask if he'd ever look at my writing. But if I asked Hank, it would take us beyond patient and nurse—into something deeper. Something I wasn't sure I was ready for.

We both started at once.

"So, my b—"

"I was thinking—"

He shifted in his seat. "Go ahead."

"No, you first," I said, my confidence wavering.

"So, I was thinking of taking my wife to Arizona," Hank continued. "She can play tennis, and I can golf all day. All the meals included. And it'll be warm."

"Sounds like your heaven."

Hank nodded, raising an eyebrow. "Well...let's not rule that destination out either," he chuckled. I couldn't help but laugh along with him.

He placed his book aside and rolled up his sleeves, ready to tell more stories. We talked about his recent visit to his son's, his Thanksgiving plans, and the family trip they had coming up for Christmas—stories that made my ribs ache from laughter.

"All set," I said, deaccessing his mediport.

"I'm done? Just like that?"

"Just like that."

Hank always lingered on his exit. Likely because he wanted to get in one more joke or story. And he always did.

"I'd like to go golf now, but I don't know if I want to deal with 'the people,' you know?" He smiled, wry.

"Wear your headphones," I joked. He once told me he wore his headphones floating under his shirt—unplugged, disconnected—so he wouldn't have to talk to "the people."

"People love the superficials," he mused. "They love to ask, 'What do you do for work?' And it's not because they want to know what I do—it's because they want to tell me what they do."

He stood, anchoring himself. "And they want to tell me all about it." His hands gestured, miming these fictitious people unloading their life stories onto him. "Who cares." He waved, as if the hypothetical crowd were beside him.

I smiled in amusement. Small talk dressed up as connection, everyone waiting for their turn to speak.

As Hank lingered, my book maintained its quiet persistence. Should I ask him?

"So, will I see you next time?" Hank asked.

"I hope so, Hank," I said with a smile, carrying the weight of the words left unspoken.

"Even a sick old man likes being picked."

I shook my head, smiling.

He hesitated, just for a second.

"All right, well—hey. I'll be in touch."

His tried-and-true exit line.

He peeled himself away.

Hank didn't like goodbyes either.

Maybe that's why he lingered.

They felt so final, sometimes.

STAGE IV

"Hank passed."

Robin's words pierced through my chest as she wrapped an arm around my shoulder.

"I know he was your buddy."

Her eyes softened when they met mine.

I opened my mouth, but nothing came out. A dull ache rose in my chest, pressing against everything I hadn't let myself feel.

"How?" I finally managed.

"Septic, I think. Here, come back with me."

Robin escorted me to the break room.

It reminded me of Brooke years ago, crying for reasons she couldn't name.

Except this time, the reason was clear.

But I couldn't cry.

I stood there, hollow. Hank was terminal from the start, but he became someone I looked forward to seeing. He brought ease, humor, and something human to the chair.

My mind reached for him in the only ways it knew. I found myself muttering pieces of our last encounter—his gait—worn, but still full of spunk, his quick wit, all the travels he had planned.

The finality settled—heavy and unyielding.

I always felt just outside the rush with Hank, lost in our own bubble of laughter: A worn treatment chair. Dingy curtains. Outdated walls. Cocktails of chemotherapy. That was all it took to forge a friendship.

"I loved his company," I murmured, my breath shallow. "He was…so funny, and he hated stupid rules as much as I did." I exhaled sharply, trying to steady myself. "I'll miss seeing him here."

Robin rubbed my shoulder. "You let him in, and that's okay."

They all cross my heart for different reasons. Some I let in. Others forget my name before they exit. Hearts are like that. They open, rush, skip, and break. I knew all along Hank would break mine. He was never curative—always terminal. But that's the thing about life—knowing doesn't soften the ache.

The familiar routine of the cancer center, despite its losses, continued. New patients arrived, treatments proceeded, and life moved forward. But there was an emptiness in the chairs and in my heart. Amid the hustle, I wondered how easily we let routine mask the weight of what we've lost.

POLLEN

No one else knew the Hank I knew in the chair. My coworkers had cared for him, but not like I had. And once I left the unit, I left them too. There was no shared memory to revisit, no stories to swap over coffee.

That's the thing about oncology grief—it's private. Unwitnessed. When a family member dies, I call someone who loved them too. We remember together. That remembering is part of the healing. But with patients, the remembering is often silent.

And then Meg called. She didn't say hello.

"I'm sorry, Duff. Hank sounded like a character. I mean, who else makes it to your funny list?"

I smiled, tears still nowhere to be found.

"He was in the number one slot for a while," I joked.

"What?" she chuckled. "He passed me?" I smiled, the kind that comes from remembering someone you're not ready to miss.

"I can't cry," I admitted. "What's wrong with me?"

There was a pause. Then her voice, dry and familiar: "Remember, we laugh so we don't cry."

"But I want to cry," I said. "I feel like I should."

"Then laugh harder," she replied. "Eventually, something leaks."

We walked together, Meg in my ear. Her voice steadied me, like it always did.

"You let him in," she said. "That's why it hurts."

"I knew he'd break my heart," I admitted.

"And you let him anyway," she said. "That's the good kind of brave."

She didn't try to fix it. She never did. She just stayed on the line long enough for me to remember that grief isn't always loud.

Sometimes it's dry-eyed.

The next morning, something gave.

And when Dave asked what was wrong,

I blamed it on the pollen.

WHAT REMAINS

I write in the silence before sunrise.

Mornings are my canvas, before the sun paints the sky and my crowd awakens. I sit in the corner of our office. Windows line one wall, and pictures of my children adorn the others. Between them hangs Nancy's welcome sign. It is a reminder that we live on.

On my nursing badge sits a guardian angel, given to all of Dean's nurses. He thought we were his angels. Maybe the truth is we end up with a few of our own.

In my scrubs pocket, I carry healing stones from a patient's husband. He hoped I could help her heal. She is alive and well today.

We still have water filters in our showers—a precaution from a patient worried about our water.

Every summer, I catch the sunrise with my children. A patient insisted I take them. They still talk about those simple mornings when the sun rose from the ocean. It's now a family tradition.

During a two-foot snowstorm, we made snow angels on the beach. Just for the wonder of it.

We still read *The City Dog and the Country Frog*. The lamb stuffie, after all its random singing, disappeared into the night.

Both hold a deeper meaning than I ever imagined.

Big Sky is our favorite skiing spot. It always will be. The connection runs deep.

I wish I could tell Ed and Maureen about our ski adventures.

Tell Nancy about the life I've built, about love and all its lessons.

I wish I could share our sunrise tradition with that patient.

Ski with Maya.

Eat at Benny's.

Do a yoga retreat with Madeline.

I wish I had written to Gail sooner.

I wish Erin's letters had grown with her children.

I wish I could hear Hank's funny stories. And that I asked him to help with mine.

But as I wish for these moments, I wonder...

Would they have existed without the urgency of time?

Would their stories have held the same weight if they weren't living like they were dying?

Within these conversations that inspired and shaped me—where I gained insight and lost judgment—lies an undercurrent of grief.

I started to notice, in my writing journey, that most of my stories were about those who lived with cancer and died from it. Cancer is no longer the automatic death sentence it once was.

People are living with cancer.

In remission.

Cancer-free.

I started to look for more stories about survivors.

I jogged my memory and skimmed my notes but came up short.

There was Siena, whose friendship outlasts hospital walls. Jolene still sends updates, telling me how she's living her life.

There was the AML patient from my early years—one of the few in my two-year inpatient stint—who, every January, posts on Facebook the anniversary of her leukemia diagnosis. She was my New Teach. I remember her eyes as clear as day—bright with hope, shadowed with trepidation. Every January, when I see her post, something catches in my chest.

She reminds me why we keep pressing forward.

Many patients stop by the clinics I've worked in over the years. They come for a follow-up appointment and pause, one foot out the door, to tell us about their lives. It's always moving to hear their stories—to see their lives unfolding because of the advancements in medicine.

People are living with diagnoses that were terminal twenty, ten, even five years ago.

Their stories are the light in a sea of darkness.

But I realized, while their stories inspire me, it's the ones who are no longer here who fill these pages.

They are the ones I carry with me.

Every day.

A WHALE'S TAIL

Over the last decade-plus, I've seen beauty unfold in people's lives simply by showing up for work. Each day, my patients remind me of what matters—the fragile beauty of existence, those fleeting moments that shimmer like the sun's first light on water.

I pause at the awe in Davey's eyes as we stand on the jetty jutting into the ocean. I feel small looking out at the horizon. At six, he must too. With its rhythmic waves, the taste of salt in the warm breeze, and the sand gripping our feet, the sea is the ultimate sensory experience.

As we stare ahead, a cloud of mist rises from the water's surface. The water erupts. A massive tail rises, catches the sunlight, and crashes back into the sea. The spray hangs in the air like stardust. It is the kind of moment that makes your world stand still.

It takes us both somewhere different than we were a moment before. Davey and I look up with smiles stretching ear to ear.

"That was a whale, Davey! We just saw a whale!"

The magic of the moment is painted across his face.

"Will he come back?" His big brown eyes are full of hope, pulling me into his world of wonder.

I watch the water, waiting.

"I hope so."

The quiet stretches between us, the water holding its breath. It reminds me of every patient I've parted ways with—the unknown stretching between us like an endless horizon. Never knowing if they would return. Only that the moment they were here mattered.

"Me too," he says, smiling.

We stand there for a few more seconds, holding onto it as long as it lets us.

The morning sun glides across the ocean, its first light illuminating the sky and water below. Davey tires of the wait and turns to climb the jetty with his siblings. I jump down to the wet sand. The surf flows up my legs, reaching my knees. A shiver travels up my spine, knocking the dust off my soul.

Dave wraps his arms around my shoulders. The cuffs on his sleeves are rolled up, his forearms spreading instant warmth. I stare into the horizon, the new light shifting across the sky. It is a breathtaking backdrop to my children's untamed shadows gliding along the jetties, leaving footprints on the sands of time.

EPILOGUE

2025—PITTSBURGH, PA

The return wasn't dramatic. No big announcement, no sense of coming full circle. Just a couple of Pods in the driveway on a sunny morning, the kids weaving between boxes, Dakota darting after squirrels again as if she'd forgotten they existed.

Pittsburgh looked the same and different all at once—the way places do when you've lived other lives in between. The hills rose and fell the way I remembered, the air carrying that familiar weight of river and rain. But I wasn't the same woman who left. I'd lived a lifetime since then, the kind that makes familiar places tilt.

Sometimes on my drive home from work, I pass the turn that once led to UPMC. I don't take it. I only notice it now, the way you notice something you put away long ago because it didn't fit anymore.

The kids are a little older now. Their backpacks bigger, their legs longer, their questions sharper. Dave still travels. Evenings still settle the same way—filled with trampoline jumps and wiffleball, catching lightning bugs in their hands before letting them go again. They live inside the moment in a way I'm finding my way back to.

And I still walk beside people. Different patients, different stories, different rooms. But the same hum of humanity. The same flashes of clarity. The same reminder that the cliff is always there, half a mile ahead, whether we look at it or not.

Maybe that's what these years have taught me—not how to outrun the cliff, but how to keep noticing the forest. How to stay awake to the small things. How to hold the moments that glow for a while and then dissolve, leaving something behind in their place.

We're home again, the six of us.

Not because the city is perfect or forever, or because the timing was right, but because this is where the next stretch of the walk lies.

And I'm still learning how to walk it—
with awareness, with gratitude,
and with the ones who let me walk beside them.

ACKNOWLEDGMENTS

To my mom, who has shown up for me in every season, steady and sure, her presence and belief carrying me farther than she knows.

To my dad, who taught me that who we become starts long before we choose it, and whose quiet curiosity still guides the way I listen, ask, and understand.

To Dave, for supporting the quiet I needed to write a book in a house full of chaos. Always without complaint. Always with a smile.

To my children, who remind me how to live wild and free, to meet the world with wonder, and to find play in the moments that move faster than I can hold them.

To the nurses on WCC7, who taught me how to be a nurse with both skill and heart.

To my MSK team on Thoracic 9, who showed me what a work environment can feel like at its best—where humor, grit, and tenderness live side by side, and where I learned how deeply a team can shape the way you move through the world.

To the nurses at the Tunnell Cancer Center, who made space for my stories before I knew what they were becoming.

To my aunts, who believed in my writing long before I ever called it that.

To Shan, whose fearless curiosity nudged me toward the places and perspectives that helped shape this book.

To Meg, for always finding the laughter and the lessons.

To Grill, for the clarity, honesty, and years of steady belief that strengthened both me and this work.

To Michelle, whose careful edits, honest guidance, and unwavering support helped me shape this book into what it became.

And to Maya, who gave me the push to stretch beyond my own edges, and whose courage and light changed me.

ABOUT THE AUTHOR

Tara Duffy is an oncology nurse and writer based in Pittsburgh, Pennsylvania. For more than a decade, she has cared for patients living at the edge of life—work that has shaped the way she sees motherhood, marriage, and the small, ordinary moments that anchor a life. She spends much of her time outdoors with her family and their retriever mix, Dakota, moving through the seasons together. *The Ones I Carry* is her debut memoir.

www.ingramcontent.com/pod-product-compliance
Lightning Source LLC
LaVergne TN
LVHW090337210926
848480LV00004B/1446